Healthy Digestion the Natural Way

Preventing and Healing Heartburn, Constipation, Gas, Diarrhea, Inflammatory Bowel and Gallbladder Diseases, Ulcers, Irritable Bowel Syndrome, Food Allergies, and More

D. LINDSEY BERKSON
with a Foreword by Jonathan Wright, M.D.

John Wiley & Sons, Inc.

New York · Chichester · Weinheim · Brisbane · Singapore · Toronto

Library of Congress Cataloging-in-Publication Data:

Berkson, Lindsey.
    Healthy digestion the natural way : preventing and healing heartburn,
  constipation, gas, diarrhea, inflammatory bowel and gallbladder diseases,
  ulcers, irritable bowel syndrome, food allergies, and more /
  D. Lindsey Berkson.
      p.   cm.
    Includes index.
    ISBN 0-471-34962-3 (paper)
    1. Indigestion—Alternative treatment. 2. Gastrointestinal
  system—Diseases—Alternative treatment. 3. Holistic medicine.
  4. Naturopathy.   I. Title.
  RC827.B467   2000
  616.3—dc21   99-32330
                                                   CIP

Printed in the United States of America

10 9 8 7 6 5

To Jonathan Wright, M.D.
For his great mind and unique heart
and for always believing in me

Contents

PART III: HOW TO FIND OUT
WHAT'S WRONG AND FIX IT

FOREWORD

For sixty years or more we have all been sold hundreds of billions of dollars of remedies for stomach and intestinal symptoms based on a series of *myths*. These myths are aggressively promoted to support product sales, but not supported by a close look at the function of our stomachs and intestines. Unfortunately, because of the emphasis on drug therapy, conventional medicine has not been motivated to purge us of these myths, but rather supports them in a lukewarm fashion.

We are sold "acid-blocking" or "acid-absorbing" medications for "acid" indigestion when the problem, more often than not, is *too little acid*. We are sold "gas pills" as if chronic excess gas were perfectly normal. We are not told that a chronic gas problem is a warning sign of a digestive malfunction that should— and can—be corrected for improved health. "Anti-spasmodic" tablets are routinely prescribed without much attention to *what* our intestines are trying to tell us with those spasms. What does "irritable bowel syndrome" mean? Shouldn't there be a reason our bowels get "irritable"?

Dr. Lindsey Berkson's book goes behind all the myths, providing a clear explanation of the complex subject of gastrointestinal health and how it relates to the health of the entire body. As she points out, it is not just "you are [physically] what you eat," but more accurately, "you are [physically] what you eat, digest, and absorb." As she explains, if absorption of the normal full range of nutrients is not happening—as is the case in nearly anyone with even mild-to-moderate gastrointestinal symptoms—*health problems can develop nearly anywhere else in the body,* caused by a lack of one or more key nutrients. A common example is fatigue; we do not realize it is often attributed to cellular malnutrition brought on by poor digestion and assimilation of nutrients. Many, many problems elsewhere in our bodies can be traced back to this single cause.

Dr. Berkson explains the normal process of digestion and details both the common and uncommon things that can and do go wrong, given "modern" food and the many stresses of modern living. She gives us complete, easy-to-follow self-help programs for correcting them without the use of all those acid blockers, antacids, gas absorbers, antispasmodics, and so on, which just cover up gastrointestinal symptoms while the rest of our health deteriorates. Instead, by actually finding and eliminating the real causes, we not only eliminate the gastrointestinal symptoms, we help improve the health of every cell in our bodies!

By now, you may have a gut feeling that this is the book about gastrointestinal health you have been looking for, more complete than you were expecting. You are right. Dr. Lindsey Berkson explains the well-known (but often overlooked) connection between "feelings" (including "gut feelings"), the intestinal tract, and the immune system. It is information you shouldn't miss. And while she is being complete—but always clear and easy to follow—she tells us about food allergies, subclinical nutrient deficiencies, detoxification, and all about the origin and healing of ulcers, inflammatory bowel disease, gallbladder disease, and many other gastrointestinal problems.

By the time you have finished this book, you will be able to see through all the massive advertising for so-called treatments for "acid indigestion," "gas," "spasms," and so on. You will be able to tell whether the remedy is truly worthwhile or nothing more than a symptom suppressor. But more important, you will have a much clearer and deeper understanding of gastrointestinal health and how it is a true key to the health of the rest of the body.

Jonathan V. Wright, M.D.
Tahoma Clinic
Kent, Washington

Acknowledgments

Many people's hard work and knowledge have been instrumental in optimizing my practice of nutrition and making it possible for me to write this book. Special thanks go to Drs. Jonathan Wright and Alan Gaby, both of whom have been my mentors and now have become colleagues and close personal friends.

Along my path, Drs. Bernard Jensen, Paavo Airola, Jeffrey Bland, David Horrobin, and Leo Galland have been teachers and now are also colleagues and acquaintances.

I also want to thank Dr. Stephen Feig, Dr. Mary James, Dr. Bob Friedman, and Sheila Lewis for their support during this process. Thanks to my editors, Tom Miller at John Wiley & Sons, Inc., and Parvati Markus. Immeasurable appreciation is due to Janet Steinberg, who, as my best friend, always makes me feel lucky. A special thanks goes to Dr. Leo Galland, who read this manuscript and recommended insightful additions.

I also want to offer my gratitude to Dr. Kevin Kopriva, who freely gave supportive health care to keep up my energy for the overwhelming challenges of this past year.

INTRODUCTION

When I first told people I was working on a book about digestive health, they usually appeared mildly interested, but felt it was nothing earth-shattering. After all, the intestinal tract is not a very sexy subject. But inevitably, they'd call later and ask if it was finished and where they could buy it. Time and time again this happened—even with people in their early twenties. Why?

Because digestive unwellness is epidemic in this country.

Most of us don't think about our digestive tract unless we have problems with it. However, millions of people have problems. Sixty-two million people a year show up in doctors' offices with digestive complaints. And this is just the number of people who go to doctors. This number does not include those who don't see doctors or who try self-help measures. *Almost half* of the adults in our country, at some time in their lives, experience intestinal illness.

There is no better substantiation of these vast numbers than a look at the best-selling drug in pharmaceutical history—the antiulcer H2 blocker Zantac. Each year its sales reach one billion dollars. This means millions of people are suffering with heartburn, stomach inflammation, and ulcers. People are taking Zantac by the truckload. Still, sales remain steadily high. Obviously, Zantac isn't making these problems go away.

Why? Because *most* drugs address the symptoms of illness, not the causes. As the sales of these drugs increase, it becomes apparent that drugs are not *curing* our intestinal illness epidemic.

Now, this isn't always true. Sometimes drugs and surgery are the best answer for particular problems. However, many times, natural answers can work as well and more safely for numerous health problems, especially digestive ones. Wisdom dictates that there are no set answers in health. What works is what works best for you with the least side effects. Any doctor or author who touts only one way to heal health problems, dogmatically supporting only one end of the spectrum, whether *holistic* (medicine emphasizing nutrition and lifestyle) or *allopathic* (traditional medicine), is to be regarded with suspicion.

But you need to learn that natural remedies such as diet, nutrients, herbs, and lifestyle changes can help alleviate most intestinal problems (emergencies excluded) before you resort to drugs. And it makes sense to try natural methods first, or at least after you have stopped pharmaceuticals, to make sure the conditions that contributed to your problem in the first place are addressed.

An example comes from one of my oldest and dearest friends. He told me that he had been having serious intestinal pains for a year. After numerous tests, the doctors had found no organic disease. With no diagnosis, they weren't offering him any treatment, so he asked me to send him some chapters of this book. Based on this information, he merely cut down the amount of food he was eating and stopped overeating late at night. He stopped abusing chocolate and caffeine and added fresh whole foods, such as unground (whole) grains and green vegetables, to his meals, along with a few nutrients.

Within two weeks, after one year of pain, and many dollars and much time spent on doctors and tests, he was pain-free. And, as an added bonus, within weeks he started to lose weight for the first time in years. He called and said, "You know, what you recommended in your book was common sense. Plain common sense. And to think no one else, neither the doctors nor I, had thought about my diet and how I was living. Thanks."

Stories like these are why I felt this book needed to be written. Now that numerous intestinal medications are being sold over the counter and we are being exposed to their multimillion-dollar advertising campaigns, we need to be aware of natural alternatives to drugs. We need to discover less expensive and safer natural remedies that may work just as well as drugs, if not better. And we need to learn to look at how we are living and eating, to figure out if our habits are the source of our problems.

Furthermore, *this book isn't just about digestive illnesses.* You might have logically thought that a book on digestive problems is *only* about digestive problems, but that isn't so. This work, while offering easy-to-grasp nutritional and lifestyle answers for numerous digestive conditions, is also a *user's manual* for everyone who eats food and needs to digest it.

We all falsely assume that just because we swallow food, we digest it. This is not true. Often what we eat is not adequately assimilated. Many of us overeat, yet our cells starve.

Inadequate digestion, or maldigestion, compromises *all* aspects of health. And symptoms of maldigestion are *not* restricted to the intestines. *Maldigestion can and does affect all other parts of your body.* Emergent medical research is demonstrating a link between inadequate digestion and numerous illnesses, ranging from allergies, headaches, and joint pains to depression, poor memory, fatigue, and more.

When I first studied with Dr. Bernard Jensen twenty years ago at his Hidden Valley Health Ranch, he taught that all health begins in the colon. My friend

Dr. Paavo Airola agreed. When I wrote my thesis for my master's degree in nutrition, the way in which overall health was linked with digestion came up time and time again.

When I did a medical-student rotation with Dr. Jonathan Wright for holistic medicine, he emphasized evaluating digestive competence when treating any disease. Both he and my other early teachers, Dr. Jeffrey Bland and Dr. Leo Galland, taught detailed methods of stool analysis to evaluate digestion, and recommended doing such analyses for most patients. As I spent literally thousands of hours over the next twenty years going through medical journals, reading and collecting massive amounts of information on health, the importance of assimilating food into the cells of the body was consistently demonstrated.

In my practice, I specialized in patients who had gone to many doctors but not gotten well. Often they had been traveling the medical circuit for years, to no avail. Most of them had ended up with doctors who told them that their health problems were all in their head. In other words, I got especially difficult cases. And, if you talk to my devoted nurse, Theo, or any of my colleagues, you will know that about 75 percent of these patients attained complete health.

I think the core of our success was the sequence of our program. We started with an initial exam and interview. For one to two hours, we gathered complete, minute details of patients' problems, family health history, what had been happening in their lives several years before things started to go bad, and their lifestyle and dietary habits. They were given a complete medical exam and a special nutritional exam that suggested which of their nutrients were deficient.

Every patient kept a chart for a week, documenting what they ate, their emotional states, sleeping habits, exercise, energy level, and bowel movements. They tested their intestinal transit time. We did a Heidelberg capsule test to assess stomach acid, and tests to rule out food allergies. When appropriate, blood tests were done to determine nutrient levels, and a comprehensive stool analysis was performed to rule out parasites and to get a complete picture of digestion.

We started with detoxification and rebuilding programs, usually a week detox and a three-week rebuilding, followed by a customized protocol that was the result of the initial comprehensive examination and testing.

After detox and rebuilding, patients could absorb nutrients more effectively. This is why I think we got so many people well who could not find help elsewhere.

When I lectured all over the country to doctors of all disciplines (roughly two to three weekends a month for almost fourteen years), they would often report that these types of health problems took an extremely long time to heal, or that they couldn't get their patients to comply with dietary changes. But I found that if treated in the order mentioned above, healing came more rapidly and thoroughly. Rarely did it take more than three months to heal even very difficult cases. There were some exceptions, but not many.

And I did not have trouble getting my patients to make these changes. They knew that I lived what I preached, so what I said had power behind it. Also, up front, I told them that if they couldn't do this program, then they shouldn't waste their money and my time, because these were the tools I had to help them help themselves. Many patients who had been labeled impossible or malingerers or hysterical were helped. I found that patients are not crazy, they just haven't yet found the right way to heal. I believe that detox and rebuilding helps the body heal itself better than just dumping nutrients and a standard program on an already overwhelmed and sick system. And it is my experience with thousands of patients that has gone into this book.

This book is about your digestive tract—the tube that extends from your mouth to the opposite end. It is, in essence, the *outside* of the world that is *inside* the middle of you. How your food successfully crosses the border, your intestinal lining, and becomes assimilated into every part of yourself, is the very stuff of which health, vitality, or predisposition to illness is made.

Your digestive tract and how well it functions serves the *totality* of your life experience—physically, mentally, and emotionally.

Thich Nhat Hanh teaches that international peace begins with each peaceful person. To be peaceful, most of us need to be healthy. May this book contribute to your personal health and peace, and beyond. Everything is, after all, connected.

D. Lindsey Berkson
Santa Fe, New Mexico

Caution! Read This First

Information to improve your life is priceless. What is offered in this book is given in the *spirit of education*. It is not meant for self-diagnosis or self-treatment.

- All matters regarding your physical health must be supervised by a medical professional.
- If you have health problems, are pregnant, or are on medication, you must check with your doctor before stopping or altering your medication, taking supplements or herbs, or initiating a new health program.
- Never take vitamin A over the recommended daily allowance (RDA) of 5,000 IU without working with a doctor.
- The dosages in this book apply to adults only. You should not self-medicate with higher dosages than the RDAs of supplements without professional supervision.

However, no one doctor catches every problem or has all the answers, so *the more you know, the more you can help your doctor(s) help you.* Never assume that a physician in authority can't make mistakes. There is such an explosion of information these days that it is not possible for any one doctor to be on top of all new research and developments. Get several opinions, educate yourself, and take responsibility.

How to Use This Book

It is possible certain individuals may suffer allergic reactions from using a natural dietary supplement or some substance mixed in with it. Call your doctor immediately if any reaction occurs. Unless you are willing to assume the risk yourself, which is part of the spirit of self-responsibility, do not use any of the information in this book.

Read the first four chapters before you look up your condition, so you understand important background material, intestinal ecology, how to take nutrients, etc.

Tools this book offers

To help you understand and use this information practically and easily, different tools are presented for each condition:

1. *Clear explanations of each condition* are presented with examples based on real-life situations (combining various patients and changing their names).
2. *Specific foods and diets* that are helpful for healing each condition are suggested for acute (one-time) and chronic (long-term) episodes of the condition.
3. *Specific juices and herbal combinations* are recommended. Juicing is one of the best ways to enjoy immediate nutritional benefits. Freshly made juices taste so good that, once you get used to them, you won't want to go back to store-bought pasteurized beverages. Freshly juiced fruits and vegetables, compared to processed juices, are like the difference in taste between vine-ripened tomatoes and commercially plastic-packed ones. Treat your family and buy a juicer; it's a worthwhile investment.
4. *Specific nutrients* are suggested. You are encouraged, *along with assistance from a doctor,* to try different combinations and find which ones work best for you. Lists of suggested nutrients are given. Try the first or second options for two weeks; if they don't work for you, go down the list and try others. *The nutrient list on page 219 gives suggestions on how to recognize low tissue levels of specific nutrients.*
5. *Reflex points* are suggested. Different organs have reflex points on various parts of the body. Stimulating these reflex points stimulates the associated organs. Using reflex points is easy to do by yourself and offers another tool of self-healing. Research has proved the effectiveness of reflexology for enhancing well-being, as well as for treating specific health problems. *Basic reflex protocol is given at the end of chapter 2 and specific points are given at the end of each chapter.*

6. *Exercises* that stimulate healing for specific digestive conditions are presented. Many of these are based on techniques I used as a yoga teacher during the fifteen years I taught classes around the country. *Basic intestinal exercises are given at the end of chapter 2 and specific exercises are given at the end of chapters.*

7. *Affirmations and meditations* are suggested for each condition. Scientific studies confirming the body-mind link are being done, especially in the arena of gastroenterology (the digestive tract). Chapter 4 succinctly explains some of this emerging information and ends with an excellent meditation that is good to do several times a week while healing any intestinal problem.

8. *Breathing exercises* assist in digestive healing, in energizing the body, and in quieting the mind. A more "silent" mind, rid of anxiety and stress, is an essential aspect of healing many digestive ailments.

Why are natural remedies desirable?

When a health situation is not an emergency, it makes sense to try natural alternatives for healing before turning to drugs and surgery. The reason is simple—drugs are not always safe. Articles in the *Journal of the American Medical Association* in 1995 demonstrated that taking drugs can and often does cause serious side effects. Doctors at Massachusetts General Hospital in Boston monitored randomly selected patients over a six-month period. Out of the 4,031 patients observed, 247 (6.5 percent) had adverse drug reactions. Of these, 1 percent were fatal, 12 percent were life-threatening, 30 percent were serious, and 57 percent were significant.

Drs. Alan Gaby and Jonathan Wright advise both laypeople and doctors: *"If doctors would use more vitamins, minerals, amino acids, herbs, and natural hormones, then they would not need to prescribe so many drugs."*

Thus, this book offers natural healing possibilities that you can discuss with your physician. These types of alternatives—ones that move us away from drugs, surgeries, and quick fixes, and get us to look at real causes of illness and their long-term solutions—are true answers to reducing health costs, complications, and numerous frustrations.

Self-responsibility is the basis of true freedom. Natural remedies are essential tools to help you take sensible responsibility. Work with doctors who are trained in using natural remedies. But never think that any one person or path has all the exact answers for you. When all is said and done, you are your best healer. No one will ever take your own health as seriously as you will.

PART I

All about Digestion

1 *Understanding Your Digestion*

This book is about natural answers to digestive problems, but it is also about the relationship between your digestive tract and your overall health. Who would have thought a book on digestion would end up pertaining to all aspects of your health—immune system, emotions, allergies, vitality, and more? Let me explain.

Your overall health can be pictured as a circle, with your digestive tract an essential triangle inside that circle.

The three points of digestion—absorption, assimilation, and elimination—are at the core of your overall health. Doctors and researchers recognize the importance of diet in health and well-being. Now the fundamental role of *absorbing* that diet is beginning to be appreciated.

Three Keys to the Digestive Process

- *Absorption* is the "dramatic" moment when food crosses from the *outside* world inside the middle of you (your intestinal tube), across your intestinal wall, and into your bloodstream.
- *Assimilation* occurs when the nutrients enter your cells.
- *Elimination* is part of the clean-up process—getting rid of waste products.

The gastrointestinal tract is one of the largest and most complicated organs in the human body. The surface area of your gastrointestinal tract is equivalent to the surface area of a tennis court.

You have heard the saying "You are what you eat." Well, this isn't really the whole story. It's not until your food is *optimally digested* that it actually becomes part of your body. So, the saying really should be "You are what you digest." Karen's story, which follows, illustrates this. But we actually can take this saying a little further: *"You are how you live, because your habits and emotions affect your digestion."*

Some examples:

Did you know that eating refined grains (white bread, white pasta, white rice, and refined flours in bakery goods) can create vitamin B deficiencies? Did

Overall Health

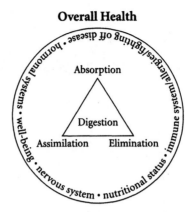

The gastrointestinal tract has the largest blood supply in the body, taking a third of the blood flow from the heart to get its job done.

you know that being low in B vitamins can promote maldigestion, or that inadequate levels of B vitamins can also make you tired, moody, anxious, or depressed?

Did you know that overconsuming alcohol stresses your ability to digest? If you drink to excess for only one evening, over the next few days a portion of the food you eat, even if it is organic and high in nutrients, could be toxic to your body rather than nourishing. Even short-term alcohol abuse can adversely affect intestinal digestion.

Emotional trauma can negatively affect digestion. It has been found that bouts of extreme anger, the loss of a loved one, or a diagnosis of catastrophic illness may adversely affect digestion for the following few weeks or even months.

KAREN'S MEMORY LOSS AND FATIGUE STARTED IN HER STOMACH

Karen was a chic, successful computer expert in Silicon Valley in northern California. At forty-two, she was happy with her job, excited by her future, but troubled by her body and mental health. She was exhausted and had significant difficulty concentrating and remembering things. After an exam and some basic blood tests, her regular physician chuckled and told her that she wasn't getting any younger.

Not satisfied, Karen asked around. A friend recommended my holistic clinic in Palo Alto. There I gave Karen an initial hour and a half interview and asked many questions, especially about her digestion. Karen said every time she ate she'd become severely bloated. Based on tests, Karen was diagnosed as having too little stomach acid, inadequate levels of B vitamins, and a diet insufficient in fiber, fresh fruits, and vegetables.

Karen was put on a nutritional program. I suggested she sit down and eat her lunch in silence and peace. After two weeks of taking digestive enzymes, eating more fruits, vegetables, whole grains, and quality protein, and doing a simple ten-minute meditation/affirmation/reflex session at home every morning, Karen was a new woman. *The key point was that Karen had not been absorbing her food optimally. She hadn't been sick enough to be diagnosed with a disease, yet she hadn't been well enough to be enjoying vitality in her life.* When she attended to her digestive tract, Karen's health returned.

Warning Signals: Red Lights on Your Body's Dashboard

If your body were a car, you'd have a dashboard. On this dashboard would be warning signals to tell you if something was wrong. Well, our bodies actually do have warning signals, but we are not trained to notice them. We often recognize illness only when we are so ill that we can no longer avoid the fact. But there were probably warning signals all along the way, if only we had noticed them. What are the warning signals that our digestion is not optimal or that we may be absorbing our food poorly?

Warning Signs of Poor Digestion	Signs of Optimal Digestion
Poor bowel habits (do not defecate daily)	Eliminate at least once a day
Frequently see undigested food in stools	Do not see undigested food in stools
Stools frequently smell foul	Stools do not smell bad
Feel better if don't eat	Feel good after eating and several
Chronic indigestion after eating	hours later
Often don't sleep well, and wake up tired	Sleep well and wake up rested

Warning Signs of Poor Digestion	Signs of Optimal Digestion
Frequently cold for no reason	Extremities (arms, legs, fingers, toes) are usually warm and have healthy pink coloring
Frequently feel "stressed," worn out, or depressed for no reason	Energy is level throughout the day
Need to loosen your belt after eating, even without overeating	Do not have extreme food cravings
Frequent burping, passing gas, and/or bloated abdomen	Do not have sudden and frequent bouts of shakiness, anxiety, depression, or anger for no reason
Pulse increases over 20 to 25 beats within 15 minutes after eating	Feel better after exercising
Chronically coated tongue	Do not have frequent mood swings

Dr. Emmanuel Cheraskin has stated that there is really only one disease: *malnutrition*. In America, many cases of malnutrition are not caused by overt starvation, but rather by eating low-quality food and doing an even lower-quality job of digesting it.

Normal vs. Abnormal Bowel Movements

The "father of medicine," Hippocrates, used to urge upon the citizens of Athens that "it was essential that they should pass large bulky motions after every meal."

People always ask me how many times a day it is normal to defecate. It's important to remember that there is a wide range of normality. However, the real question becomes: Is what is considered normal actually too wide a range, so that many people who are *abnormal* are included?

Medical textbooks say normal defecation in suburban America ranges from two to three times a day to several times a week. In my experience with thousands of people, I have found that not eliminating daily is associated with a higher risk of incurring many intestinal as well as other health problems. I have observed that when people balance their diets and nutrients enough to eliminate their symptoms of ill health, they usually have bowel movements one to three times a day.

You should eliminate *at least once a day.*

Note: Microscopic stool analyses can assess a number of facts about absorption. These tests are available through various labs. See appendix B.

Home Assessment of Digestion

Analysis of Your Stool. Good digestion should result in stools that are large, round, medium to dark brown, do not float, are not bubbly, are somewhat soft and mushy, and do not frequently exhibit undigested food. You should not need to strain. Passing stools should not hurt or burn, nor should they have a noxious odor.

Intestinal Transit Time. This is an important and easy test to do at home. Optimal digestion includes optimal intestinal transit time—the average time food takes to go through (transit) your body. Healthy intestines contract about 12 times a minute, which propels food on its digestive journey. This should optimally add up to about 24 to 30 hours from mouth to rectum. In the United States, the normal transit time is about 48 hours or larger. This is *normal,* but by no means, *optimal.* To test your transit time, use a "color marker," such as activated charcoal or corn kernels.

What to do: Swallow about 20 grains of activated charcoal tablets (5 to 12, depending on how large they are) all at once with water. You can purchase charcoal tablets from your drugstore or health-food store. If they are not available, swallow 4 tablespoons of whole corn kernels. Note the time you swallow the charcoal or corn. Then note the *first* time you see your stool turn black (from the charcoal) or you notice clumps of the corn kernels in the stool.

Optimal transit time is approximately 24 hours. With prolonged transit time, you first see indicators at 30 to 40 hours or more. If you first see indicators at 78 hours, or you never see them, this suggests a "toxic" bowel. Also, once you notice the indicators, you should keep noticing pieces of them for no more than another 12 hours. If you continue to see bits of the indicators for several more days, this is another sign of a sluggish bowel.

When I was in practice, over 20 percent of the people who took this test never saw the indicators come out. This suggested too long an intestinal transit time and a "sluggish" intestine. Not adequately eliminating waste products increases the risk of numerous diseases, as well as suffering with poor digestion.

Redo this easy home test once a year to make sure you are "on target" with optimal gastrointestinal health.

Daily Ways to be Extra Good to Your Intestines

1. What you do first thing in the morning makes a difference to your intestinal and overall health. Even if you drink coffee in the morning, at least do something nice for your intestines before the coffee hits your stomach. First thing, on rising, drink two glasses of quality filtered water.
2. Do something good for your intestines midmorning or afternoon.
   - Have yogurt with applesauce.
   - Have a piece of fruit and/or sip green tea.
   - Sit and breathe deeply, look at the sky, and have a moment of peace. This is food for your intestines, too.
3. Eat and drink healthily.
   - Eat two or three different-colored *vegetables and fruits* a day.
   - Consume at least two high-fiber foods a day (see chapter 2).
   - Drink 5 to 8 glasses of quality fluids daily. Drink *filtered or spring water*. If you eat generous amounts of fresh fruits and veggies, you can drink less. Even tea and coffee contribute (we retain half as water). On the other hand, sugary drinks such as colas are dehydrating.
4. What you do right before bed affects your health.
   - Have a glass of filtered water.
   - Sit for a moment in bed and remember one good thing from your day. Feel gratitude. Gratitude is food for your intestines, too.

Children and Digestion

Dr. Jonathan Wright, M.D., internationally renowned nutritional expert, suggests we never have a guarantee of good digestion or absorption, no matter what our age. He has records of more than fifty children under the age of three who had no outright disease, yet had inadequate digestion and absorption as proven by laboratory tests.

DAVID—BETTER LIVING THROUGH IMPROVED ABSORPTION

Seven-year-old David suffered from severe asthma. He had been diagnosed as emotionally unstable and had been seeing a psychotherapist for over a year, as well as taking drugs, but his asthma continued to worsen. David's mother took him to a nutritionally oriented doctor who discovered David had frequent tummyaches and excessive intestinal gas. Tests showed that David didn't make enough stomach acid. The doctor explained that David had not been adequately digesting his food. The undigested food particles traveled through David's body, probably causing inflammation and irritation in his lungs, contributing to his asthma and food allergies.

Within one week of taking digestive supplements and going off milk and wheat, David's stomachaches went away. Within one month the asthma was gone. David was happier and more emotionally stable. David's digestive problem was causing his asthma. Avoiding milk and wheat products and taking digestive supplements allowed David to live a normal life without dependency on steroids.

Wouldn't you want to know if your child could get rid of or improve asthma (and other problems) through diet and digestive enzymes rather than through medication? Doesn't it make sense to try natural methods first?

Optimal Digestion Needs Supportive Players

Digestion is a transformative act. It takes external matter (food) and attempts to break it down to absorbable pieces, so that some is let into the body and the rest is removed. Food kept in the body has to be broken down sufficiently to lose its *foreignness*. This lets the body accept the food as nutrition, rather than fight it as it would a foreign invader. In this sense, digestion is part of our *unifying* relationship with the external world.

There's a lot involved: from simple unsophisticated activities, such as chewing, to involved and complicated substances, such as the protective, paintlike coating of the intestinal wall. There are digestive enzymes, fiber foods, quality water, the balance between stressor foods and protector foods, the intestinal ecology (composed of friendly and unfriendly bacteria), exercise, the presence or absence of infectious agents, nutrient levels, and the health of the intestinal lining. We will talk first about the intestinal lining.

Key Functions of a Healthy Intestinal Lining

When the intestinal lining is healthy, it assists in the digestion of carbohydrates, proteins, and fats, and acts as a *traffic guard*, or *discerning barrier*, not allowing potentially noxious substances into your body (while still letting in the "good" ones). Remember, whatever substances get inside your intestinal tube are "outside" of you until they cross your intestinal lining. The lining also has an *immune* function—protecting you against and neutralizing unfriendly bugs, microorganisms, and allergic substances.

The intestinal lining has a *muscular* layer, and like any muscle, it can have good or bad tone. A weak muscular lining doesn't propel food through your intestinal tract at a healthy rate. An overstimulated muscular lining can cause spasms.

A healthy intestinal lining is *self-cleaning* and *renewing*. Because the lining of the gastrointestinal tract comes into contact with so many different foods and substances and because it has such diverse jobs to perform, it must be able to "clean and rebuild" itself quickly in order to stay competent. The cells that make up the lining of your intestinal tract are shed and replaced every three to six days. This is one of the fastest cellular turnover times (mitosis) in the human body. Because of this fast growth rate, the cells making up the lining of the digestive tract are extremely sensitive to daily nutrition, easily damaged by dietary and lifestyle indiscretions, and affected by the balance between *protector* and *stressor* factors.

Protectors of the Intestinal Lining

- *Quality food,* such as unground grains, fresh vegetables, fruits, seeds, and nuts (organic, as much as possible).
- *Vitamins and minerals and certain amino acids,* such as B complex (especially B_1, B_6, and folic acid); vitamins A, C, D, and E; zinc, selenium, manganese, molybdenum, magnesium, and arginine all nourish the intestinal lining.

How to Take Nutrients

Since nutrients are recommended for each condition discussed in this book, a short word on how to take them is essential.

Take fat-soluble nutrients (they often come in gel capsules) with fatty meals. Water-soluble nutrients can be taken at any time of day, but most people tolerate nutrients better with some food in their belly. If you have intestinal discomfort, take them throughout the meals.

It is a good idea to add one supplement a day to let your body acclimate to taking nutrients, or to identify ones that may not agree with you. Sometimes taking nutrients with digestive enzymes for the first two weeks helps you acclimate a little more easily. Take most herbs on an empty stomach 15 to 20 minutes before meals.

Whenever a separate *B vitamin* is recommended, take it with a B complex and only take the specific B vitamin for one to three months. Multiple nutrients are part of any healing program—but these programs are for limited periods of time.

- *Glutamine,* an amino acid, has a trophic, or positive growth effect on the intestinal lining. It is easily converted into 6-carbon glucose (the sugar the body uses), so it is a good intestinal fuel source for quick energy to the cells that line the intestinal tract. In this way, glutamine indirectly helps support many functions of the intestinal tract.

  The bodies of most healthy folks make plentiful amounts of glutamine from skeletal and lung muscle. In metabolically stressed individuals, such as the elderly, this manufacturing system can be overwhelmed. One reason elderly people have thinner intestinal linings is that they have less muscle mass and lung power to assist in the manufacturing of glutamine. This can be improved through exercise, which rebuilds muscle mass and lung capacity.

  Glutamine is so protective to the intestinal tract that when it is given along with chemotherapy, it reduces some of the negative side effects on the gut and enhances the overall well-being of the cancer patient, as well.

- *Flavonoids* are found in more than 4,000 widely occurring plant foods, especially the leaves or outer parts of fruits and vegetables. Flavonoids help "tighten" the junctions of the intestinal lining to assist in the important barrier function. Flavonoids give foods like wine, apples, blueberries, and blackberries their color. Flavonoids are found in most fruits, especially in apples, grapes, and berries; in vegetables like lettuce, onions, endive, broad beans, and red peppers; as well as in black and green tea, red wine, and apple juice. They are so protective of the lining of the intestinal tract that certain concentrated forms of flavonoids are used to treat stomach ulcers, allergies, and inflammation.

- *High-fiber foods* "brush" and "clean" intestinal lining cells, whereas low-fiber diets (junk food) lack this maintenance-cleaning action. Cereals and beans, high in fiber, are also high in phytic acid, which helps protect the intestinal lining. Phytic acid is found in grains and protects the colonic cells from cancerous changes.

- *Muscle tone* in the intestinal tract helps propel food (a process called peristalsis).

- *Bowel movements,* at least once a day.

- *Water* that is free from contaminants, in adequate amounts.

- *Short chain fatty acids (SCFAs)* are another growth stimulator to the intestinal lining. They supply fuel for the cells that line the colon, as well as stimulate enzymes that assist in digestion. Eating a quality diet feeds the bacteria that make SCFAs, which in turn feed intestinal lining cells.

- *Friendly bacteria,* like the *L. acidophilus* found in yogurt, help make SCFAs.
- *N-acetylglucosamine,* a nutrient made of a simple sugar and an amino group, is an essential part of the "coat" worn by all the body's cell. Studies now show it helps grow cartilage, and it also protects the intestinal lining.

Stressors of Your Intestinal Lining

- *Food stressors: Excessive* consumption of nutrient-poor foods: sugars, refined carbohydrates (white flour products like pastries, pastas, and cookies), alcohol, caffeinated beverages (black tea, colas, and coffee), table salt, saturated animal fats; *excessive* intake of animal foods, hydrogenated and processed oils; overeating of processed foods; and overeating in general.

  In other words, coffee first thing every morning, tea and cola throughout the day, along with frequent consumption of foods like doughnuts and pastries, over time will erode the intestinal lining.
- *Lifestyle stressors* are anything that disrupts the normal intestinal environment, such as surgery, chronic stress, or illness.
- *Various stressors.* Regular use of aspirin (even enterically coated) and anti-inflammatory drugs (nonsteroidal anti-inflammatory drugs—NSAIDs); infections with viruses, bacteria, and parasites; food allergies; chronic constipation or diarrhea; overgrowth of unfriendly bacteria; and nutrient deficiencies due to a variety of causes such as allergies, poor eating habits, poor exercise habits, illnesses, surgery, and trauma.
- *Developmental stress periods,* such as infancy, pregnancy, and aging, may cause more stress and demands on the intestinal environment. Environmental contamination in water, food, and air may be disruptive factors.

Intestinal Immune System

Every time you eat, your intestinal tract is exposed to a wide variety of substances, food, and microorganisms. To deal with this challenge, the intestinal tract has one of the most powerful immune systems in the body. Eighty percent of the body's lymph nodes (the immune system's hotels for white blood cells that fight off foreign invaders) are located around the intestinal tract.

Secretory IgA, protective proteins that fight off foreign invaders and substances, make a sticky *antiseptic paint* that forms a protective coating along your intestinal tract. The antiseptic paint "licks" the bad guys (toxic and allergic substances). This licking "warns" the rest of the body.

Four Factors That May Tax the Immune System of the Gut

1. Eating *excessive* amounts of refined sugar on a daily basis.
2. Eating refined (processed and hydrogenated) oils on a daily basis.
3. Eating the same foods over and over again (*repetitive eating*).
4. Eating foods you are allergic to (you may not be aware of these).

The combined actions of absorption, assimilation, elimination, and immunity are supposed to make sure that whatever gets into your bloodstream from your intestinal tract will cause as few problems as possible for the rest of your body. Avoiding *stressful* foods assists this process.

Are You Confused about What to Eat?

I think it is important to make a comment about what constitutes an optimal diet. This is because nutrition is confusing, even to experts (if they are honest). For example, one day the results of research say eggs are good, then after more studies they say eggs are bad, and then they say eggs are fine if eaten in moderation. One day fiber is protective against colon cancer and lowers cholesterol, then, with the next new study, its benefits are nil or questionable.

What is an ordinary person to do? You can't go wrong if you stay moderate. *A moderate, sensible, and optimal diet includes fresh vegetables, fruits, cultured foods like yogurt, nuts, whole grains, along with quality proteins such as beans, fish, and eggs.*

Don't believe what just one authority says. Read information from many sources and, when looking toward diet as a therapeutic tool, explore what works best for your unique body and lifestyle.

Helpful Tips

- Fresh foods: Eat many raw foods, as well as fresh vegetables cooked immediately before eating.
- Eat some fresh fruits and raw vegetables each day.
- Eat more fresh foods than commercially processed foods. Avoiding processed foods can get tricky. Many of us, for example, are eating more turkey and less red meat. But turkey in the plastic package (even in the deli section) has additives and is processed.

When I lived in Australia, any time I got a chicken or turkey sandwich, they pulled the meat right off the bones. Try to avoid processed foods as much as possible.

- Excessive consumption of processed, canned, and "dead" foods depletes health and digestive vitality. Food with long shelf life got that way from processing the life-promoting essential oils and nutrients out of it.

Not All Oils Are Created Equal

Eliminate as much processed and hydrogenated oil as possible from your diet. Look at the pressing dates on oils that need to be refrigerated to make sure you are getting a fresh product.

Try alternating oils: olive, hazelnut, flax, and sesame. Keep them tightly closed and refrigerated. Break a capsule of vitamin E into each bottle when you first open it to preserve the oil. This is because oil gets oxidized when we leave an opened bottle on the counter for a while, and toxic substances form in the oil that may have irritating effects on the intestinal lining. Since oil is fat and chemicals such as pesticides store in fat, try to buy *organic* oils whenever possible.

When you start adding tablespoons of oil to your diet, or more seeds and nuts, make sure to *take daily vitamin E orally to prevent oxidative stress from the oils.*

Mindful Eating Tips to Enhance Digestion

- Prepare an enjoyable atmosphere. Light some candles, set a nice table, sit down, and look out the window. Mealtime should be a minivacation.
- Pay attention to what you are doing. You are eating. You are feeding your body. Smell the food, see the food, enjoy the food. This enhances digestion.
- Eat in a relaxed atmosphere. Do not eat when angry, upset, or hurried. Emotional upsets disturb digestion, no matter how pure the food is.
- Eat at a moderate pace. Do not inhale your food; chew your food mindfully. This creates more self-respect and peace inside your body as well as in your digestive tract.
- Avoid drinking ice-cold drinks, or drinking too much liquid with meals. Ice-cold drinks slow down digestion and too many beverages overload digestion. Drink alcohol moderately.

Three Easy and Tasty Juices That Feed Your Intestines

Ginger cooler   Juice carrot and Granny Smith or Macintosh apple together with a slice of fresh ginger, and dilute with water to reduce sugar.

Intestinal Freshener   Juice celery, cucumbers, and carrots. Optional: Add a little mint through the juicer.

Berry Madness   Blend blueberries and strawberries with a little apple juice, some water, and protein powder. Yum. Optional: add yogurt.

Drink juices immediately. Naturally occurring enzyme activity is released by the juicing or blending and remains at its highest level for about five minutes. If vegetables and fruits have been refrigerated until right before juicing, the cool juice is even more refreshing and tasty.

Overeating

Another way to use your head is to learn to eat the right amount of food. Overeating and oversnacking are the downfall of many of us. Eat to a comfortable point, so your stomach is not stuffed. Eat only when your stomach is empty and you're really hungry. This greatly improves digestion.

Overeating is a burden on the entire digestive system. Eating too much irritates the delicate cells that line the intestinal tract. Overeating contributes to undigested food and toxins burdening the intestinal tract, the liver, and the entire body.

If you travel to Europe, one thing that will strike you is that people eat at mealtimes and rarely snack. Here in the United States, people eat in their cars, while walking, and while hanging out. We are munching and snacking all the time—we are obsessed with instant gratification. This traumatizes the digestive system and greatly contributes to many digestive ailments, as well as to other health problems.

Seven Ways to Reduce Eating Without Starving

1. Eat more unrefined whole grain products.
2. Avoid refined sugars and overeating of simple carbohydrates.
3. Have a fiber cocktail midmorning (see chapter 2).
4. Chew food twenty times before swallowing.
5. Wait ten minutes after finishing the first plate before you think about having seconds. Your satiety center needs a few minutes to kick in.
6. While you're waiting, breathe deeply several times. Think about your body and how you feel in it.
7. Rotate your foods: attempt to eat a wide variety of types and colors of foods.

It's not infrequent dietary indiscretions that matter. It's how you eat most of the time that counts.

2 Fiber, Water, and Intestinal Exercises: Secrets to Healthy Digestion

Can you guess who the first doctor was to prescribe fiber? Hippocrates, in 430 B.C. He recommended fiber to prevent constipation.

When was the last time a doctor asked you about the fiber content of your diet?

Fiber—Nature's Own Residue

What is fiber? It is the part of plant food that passes through your small intestine undigested. In other words, fiber is *residue* left over from what is digested. This is why high-fiber foods are often called high-residue foods. There are seven types of fiber, some which bind water to the stool, and others which are acted upon by intestinal bacteria to form healthful acids or miscellaneous gases.

Health-Giving Examples of High-Fiber Foods
- Whole grains (cereals, brown rice, whole rye, whole or rolled oats, oat grits, millet, buckwheat, quinoa, amaranth, whole corn, spelt, whole wheat or wheat berries). The *best* fiber is from unground (whole) grains.
- Breads, cereals, muffins, and rolls made from whole grain flour.
- Raw fruits, such as apples, with the skins on, and dried fruits (apricots, figs, peaches, prunes, raisins, and dates). Note: Try to use organic dried fruit as much as possible. Dried nonorganic raisins, according to FDA reports, were found to contain high levels of toxic chemicals. Apparently, pesticides, fungicides, and other chemicals get concentrated in the drying process.
- Raw or slightly cooked vegetables. Cellulose is broken down if over-cooked and then is not effective.
- Husks or skins (not shells) of seeds and nuts—best raw.

- All nuts, beans, peas, lentils, potatoes, and yams—well washed and *with their skins on.*

Processed grains and pasta—even products colorful from added vegetables—along with white bread, white rice, white pasta, refined grains and flours, and animal foods such as meats and eggs, are *devoid* of fiber.

TUMMYACHES IN CHILDREN LINKED TO LOW FIBER

Seven-year-old Tommy had a quick mind and had started an innovative hobby. Monthly, he wrote up a one-page paper about the folks in his neighborhood. But one month Tommy didn't get the paper done. He was suffering with one of his chronic stomachaches.

A neighbor told Tommy's mother she had read that a common cause of tummyaches in young children was insufficient fiber in the diet. So Tommy's mom started to cook him whole-grain cereals plus lots of vegetables. She bought him bran muffins and even cookies with added bran. By the next month, Tommy was pain-free and the neighbors were enjoying reading about themselves in his paper once again.

Not All Fiber Is the Same

Different fibers act differently. They differ in how they hold water. Thus, fibers are classified according to their water solubility.

Insoluble fibers hold less water than soluble fibers. Whole wheat is an example of insoluble fiber. It holds only *three times* its weight in water. Types of insoluble fibers are cellulose, some hemicellulose, and lignins. Translated into food, this means whole grains, vegetables, and most brans. Insoluble fibers provide the *bulk* of the stool and help maintain healthy stool transit time. Insoluble fibers have many other beneficial effects; for example, wheat bran and flaxseed help maintain optimal levels of estrogen in the body.

Soluble fibers hold much more water than insoluble fibers. They are natural gel-forming fibers. These hold *forty times* their weight in water. Soluble fibers are the primary food source for friendly bacteria in the intestinal tract. Friendly bacteria act on the fiber and produce short-chain fatty acids. SCFAs make an acid environment and protect and feed a healthy colon.

Soluble fiber comes from psyllium, legumes, beans, and oats. These are good foods to eat, especially if you are at risk for colorectal diseases such as hemorrhoids or cancer.

Decreased soluble fiber in the diet leads to constipation, reduced growth of friendly bacteria, growth of abnormal or unfriendly bacteria, less healthy cells in the lower portion of the colon, increased risk of colorectal cancer, and an excessively alkaline pH in the lower portion of the colon.

Other fibers are *pectins* from apples and citrus, which hold *one hundred times* their weight in water. Pectins protect the colon against cancer. Quality fiber supplements offer you several types of fibers.

Most Americans eat about 12 grams of fiber a day. To give an example, one apple has about one gram of fiber. The National Cancer Institute recommends eating an average of 25 grams of fiber a day (20 to 30 grams is a good range).

Seven Tasty Soluble Fiber Treats

1. Grated apples over oatmeal made from whole oats.
2. Grated apples mixed into yogurt. Optional: Add low-fat granola.
3. Grated pear over yogurt, kefir, or even vanilla ice cream or healthy ice-cream substitutes.
4. Apple slices with cheese.
5. Handful of nuts and dried fruit.
6. Brown rice and vegetables.
7. Whole-wheat tortilla filled with vegetables and avocado.

Benefits of Eating Fiber

During World War II, Denmark stopped refining flour for economic reasons. When the population was forced to eat whole flour and thus more fiber, the death rate went down and there was a marked decline in cancer, heart disease, diabetes, and high blood pressure.

Why did the Danes do so well eating unrefined grains? Because fiber performs so many beneficial functions for the body.

Fiber helps prevent and heal a wide variety of gastrointestinal problems such as peptic ulcers, irritable bowel syndrome, hiatal hernias, inflammatory bowel diseases, gallbladder disease, and even hemorrhoids. Insufficient fiber contributes to 25 percent of digestive disorders.

Fiber keeps the waste material inside your intestines soft and bulky, taking pressure off your muscular intestinal tube and preventing hernias. This also prevents diverticular disease (see page 88). Fiber *brushes* the cells that line your intestinal tract to keep them healthy. This optimizes nutrient absorption and indirectly benefits immune function.

Fiber normalizes the time food takes to go through the body and, in this way, protects and treats many cases of constipation and diarrhea, and also helps maintain an optimal balance of friendly bacteria.

Higher-fiber diets reduce sugar craving, thus indirectly preventing dental cavities. Fiber is also helpful in protecting against varicose veins, diabetes, heart disease, appendicitis, and certain food-coloring toxicities.

Fiber and Blood Sugar: Promoting Optimal Body Weight

Fiber slows the absorption of carbohydrates, which then slows down the release of insulin. This is a vitally important aspect of fiber. Quick release of insulin and abnormal elevations of insulin, called insulin "spiking," are being connected to a wide variety of health problems such as elevated cholesterol and triglycerides, low protective cholesterol (HDL), heart disease, diabetes, and even certain cancers such as breast cancer.

Eating sugary foods without sufficient fiber causes your blood sugar and insulin to elevate. What goes up must come down. After eating sugary low-fiber foods like doughnuts in the morning, there is a *reactive* low blood sugar phenomenon later in the day, often experienced as the afternoon "slump." Fiber foods, on the other hand, help stabilize blood sugar by slowing down the release of sugars and insulin. This reduces the highs and lows of sugars and insulin. In this way, fiber foods protect against risk factors for diabetes, and help maintain optimal energy throughout the day.

Fiber also protects against obesity by helping to promote a sense of satiety, a contented feeling of "fullness" from a normal amount of food. Eating a breakfast that includes whole grains helps prevent the urge to binge and overeat later in the day.

Note: Some sensitive people (with Syndrome X) react to certain carbohydrates, such as breads (even whole-grains breads) in a similar way to sugars (see Carbohydrate Warnings later in this chapter).

Fiber reduces cholesterol. It does this by preventing reabsorption of bile acids in the intestinal tract. This makes the liver convert more cholesterol into bile acids and lowers the cholesterol level in the blood. This is good for your heart, intestinal tract, immune system, and gallbladder.

Fiber and Women

Some friendly bacteria act on fiber and make substances that appear to protect against excessive or imbalanced estrogen conditions such as PMS, painful (fibrocystic) breasts associated with menstruation, infertility, and breast cancer. Insufficient fiber promotes an environment where certain bacteria can promote recirculation of estrogen, which may aggravate these types of problems.

Some studies have shown that constipation is associated with a higher risk for abnormal breast cells.

Fiber and Colon Cancer

Since the 1960s, it has been observed that Western countries with diets lowest in fiber have the highest rates of colon cancer in the world, and that native African populations who eat high-fiber diets have lower incidence rates of this cancer. Numerous studies have suggested a protective effect from fiber, but two Harvard studies, in 1994 and 1999, found no protective link between fiber and colorectal cancer. However, the levels considered to be high-fiber consumption in these studies are being questioned by some experts. Even though study results seem to zigzag, it is still considered prudent to consume a diet higher in vegetables, fruits, and grains and lower in fried meats (darkened on the surface). Don't despair at the way science works; it usually takes decades to figure out true cause and effect. Fiber is still a good guy.

The Fiber Cocktail

Easy Fiber Cocktail

Add one heaping teaspoon of some kind of bran, usually psyllium (or oat, soy, or rice bran) to an 8 oz. glass of water or diluted fruit juice. Stir briskly and drink quickly, and follow with a second glass of plain water.

Or, swallow two fiber tablets and drink one to two large glasses of water.

Take once or twice a day one-half hour before or two hours after meals so as not to inhibit absorption of nutrients.

Rotate your fiber source to avoid eventually forming allergic reactions. You can become allergic to anything you take on a daily basis, especially if it is processed (as fiber sources are). So if you take fiber daily, buy two or three sources and rotate them. If you take fiber and become constipated for several days, develop canker sores, a sore mouth or tongue, allergic shiners (dark circles under your eyes), or develop new symptoms, you may be allergic to the source.

It's a good idea to take a fiber cocktail one to three times a week, even if you already eat a balanced diet high in fiber foods. This is because not all fiber is "equal," and it's extremely difficult to regulate how much you get.

Taking too much fiber too quickly can give you gas, diarrhea, or even, surprisingly enough, can cause constipation for a day or two. So start *slowly*.

What Do You Get When You Eat Refined Fiber-Deficient Foods?

You get less quality protein. Quality protein is a normal protector of the stomach lining. Eating refined grain, which has less quality protein, makes the stomach more vulnerable to normal amounts of stomach acid and may contribute to stomach ulcers and inflammation (gastritis). Refined carbohydrates are metabolized in your body like sugars. Eating these foods actually increases your sugar burden and uses up precious vitamins and minerals. All this may increase your risk of stomach ulcers as well as health problems.

Refined grains also produce harder stools, as less water is held in your intestines. This puts more pressure on the muscular wall of your intestines, which increases the risk of diverticular disease (weakened pouches of intestinal muscle that can affect digestion and get inflamed).

You get less spark of life in your food and less flavor. Once you get used to the taste of whole grains, refined grains taste inferior. And you miss out on a free reflexology treatment each day. (High-fiber foods have been *theorized* to stimulate reflex points along the intestinal tract.)

Carbohydrate Warnings!

- Some people mistakenly add more refined high-carbohydrate foods to their diet when they try to increase their fiber. Misinformed, they purchase foods like spinach noodles, thinking these are whole foods. Wrong. Pasta needs to be made from whole grains to be a whole-food source. White flour with added green vegetables, like most green pasta, doesn't count. Read the label. It should state the grains are "whole."
- The emphasis is on *unprocessed*. Cereals, even high-fiber ones, high-fiber breakfast bars, and other commercially advertised products are still processed. They are better than refined grains, but not as good as consuming plain whole grains.
- Commercial high-fiber products often contain excess sugars (from fruit, dates, honey, fructose, etc.). This puts a sugar burden on the body and the intestinal lining.
- It has been estimated that one-third of the population needs to eat a healthy balance between high-carbohydrate food sources and adequate proteins. This is because certain people are genetically predisposed to oversecrete the sugar-lowering hormone insulin when they consume large or even moderate amounts of carbohydrates, even those from grains, fruits, and juices, as well as from refined sugars. A fair number of people probably have a hard time shedding pounds, even though they eat salads and exercise, because eating too many high-density carbohydrates—such as grains, starches, pasta, pastries—causes them to hypersecrete insulin. These people still need some high-fiber, high-carbohydrate foods. But they should not overconsume them. And they must be careful to make sure they consume adequate protein.

The tendency to secrete excess insulin has been labeled *Syndrome X*. You are at risk for Syndrome X if your parents or grandparents were diabetic, had heart disease, elevated cholesterol or triglycerides, or carried extra weight around the waist for much of their lives. In a person prone to Syndrome X, high-glycemic foods are more likely to bump up blood sugar and insulin levels. This is not healthy. People with Syndrome X may also be at greater risk for some types of cancers.

If you are at high risk for Syndrome X, try the following:

Add high-fiber food sources into your diet carefully. Do not overeat refined goodies, grains, fruits, fruit juices, potatoes, or carrots. Eat adequate protein along with meals containing high-fiber, high-carbohydrate foods. Whole rye and oats are your best grains. Apples are your best fruits. For further information, read *The Zone Diet* (Sears) and *Protein Power* (Eades and Eades). Ask your doctor to run both fasting and postprandial (two hours after eating) insulin blood tests.

Remember, an optimal diet is one that's in harmony with your genetic makeup.

NOTE: An unusual disease called *systemic sclerosis* affects the entire gastrointestinal tract. People with this disease should *avoid* a high-fiber diet, as it can be dangerous for them. Also, one study shows that fiber supplementation in some *diabetics* may inhibit the absorption of vitamin A, so diabetics should be monitored, especially children. However, in this study, high amounts of supplemental fiber were given *with* lunch and dinner, rather than separate from meals.

Glycemic Index

Glycemic index refers to the rate at which carbohydrates enter the bloodstream. The lower the rate, the less this food adversely affects blood-sugar and insulin release. The following information is adapted from Dr. Barry Sears's *Enter the Zone.* If you think you could be prone to Syndrome X, make more food choices from list 1 than from list 2.

1. Low and moderate glycemic-rate food choices

Yogurt, eggs, turkey, chicken, soybean products, most beans, apples, applesauce, pears, peaches, grapes, cherries, grapefruits, plums, green vegetables, whole oats, whole-grain cereals, whole-grain rye bread, barley, milk, ice cream, fructose, and nuts.

2. High glycemic-rate food choices

White bread, white rice, puffed-rice cakes, highly sugared breakfast cereals, millet, French bread, whole-wheat bread, brown rice, maltose sugar, corn chips, carrots, corn, bananas, raisins, figs, dates, apricots, instant potatoes, instant rice, sugar from malt, and low-fat or soy or rice ice creams.

Easy Ways to Get More Fiber into Your Diet

Sprouted grains are good fiber sources. They are less acidic than nonsprouted grains, which is good because an alkaline-based diet is desirable. Sprouts contain the germ, or the reproductive power, that has the vitality to grow the next generation—to perpetuate life.

Your health-food store sells a wide variety of sprouted-grain breads, muffins, even tortillas and bagels. If your grocery store or co-op doesn't have these items, ask the manager to order them. Alvarado Bakery has a complete line. My favorites are their onion and poppy-seed bagels. They even have sprouted spelt bagels. Manna breads are sprouted, taste like cake, and are wonderful warmed up with a little butter, oil, cottage cheese, fruit spread, or just plain. They make unique breakfasts or snacks and are sold at most health-food stores. Sprouted breads with carrots, raisins, and nuts can be served like cakes.

Tasty Sprouted-Grain Treats

- Toasted onion or poppy-seed bagel with yogurt, sliced red onion, a slice of turkey or smoked salmon and tomato.
- Butter (raw, organic, and salt-free tastes exceptionally great) with fruit spread on spelt bagels.
- Scrambled or poached egg on sprouted bagel or bread.
- Manna bread, warmed under the broiler, with almond butter or cottage cheese and sugar-free fruit spread.
- Sprouted tortillas with melted cheese (soy, goat, or cow) and a handful of sprouts and minced onions.
- For dessert, warm cut-up fruit-and-nut sprouted breads, topped with melted cheese or natural sweets like frozen yogurt or rice or soy ice-cream substitutes.

Sprouted-Bean Delights

Bean sprouts are high in fiber, nutrients, and essential oils.
- Sprinkle sprouted bean mixes (mung, lentil, and adzuki beans) on salads or in soups.
- Place sprouted beans over lunch meat inside sandwiches.
- Make easy and fast sprout salads with a mixture of sprouted beans and sunflower, and daikon radish sprouts (these are spicy, so be sparing). Add granulated garlic, olive oil, and balsamic vinegar. Optional: Add soy sauce.
- Broccoli sprouts are high in fiber and may protect against breast cancer. Wrap some inside turkey slices smeared with mustard and horseradish (especially the red kind with added beets). Yum.

Nuts and seeds are also high in fiber. Healthy and tasty seeds are pumpkin, sunflower, flax, and sesame seeds. Tahini, a sesame butter, is great in dressings and sauces. Grind flaxseeds in a coffee grinder and add to yogurts, salads, and soups.

Nuts should be eaten raw. If you don't like them raw, mix raw nuts in with toasted nuts, such as tamaried almonds. Don't get monotonous with your nuts. Try almonds, hazelnuts (filberts), pine nuts, walnuts, and pecans. Almonds, hazelnuts, macadamia nuts, and pecans have a fair amount of monosaturated fats, the same healthy fats found in olive oil.

Note: Seeds and nuts are almost half fat, so don't overeat. Many people think that if it's health food, it isn't fattening. This is not true.

Water to the Rescue

Most of us don't drink enough water. Water optimizes digestion. Here's how:

- Water has capillary action. This unique ability of water to flow against gravity allows the blood, which is 83 percent water, to complete its circuit all around your body, and helps minerals and vitamins get into cells.
- Water flushes toxins out of the body.
- Water helps the bowel have enough fluid for optimal transit time, helping to avoid the creation of cancer-causing substances in the bowel.
- Water helps elimination, which makes your skin fresher, softer, and clearer.

Myths about Water

It's *not* true that we need exactly eight glasses of water a day—if we drink other beverages and consume a sensible amount of fresh fruits and vegetables. We retain *half* the fluid from coffee or tea as water in our body. Thus, the myth that coffee and tea dehydrate (as highly sugared drinks do) isn't true. Drink two glasses of water upon rising and one before bed, along with several glasses a day besides other beverages, unless your activity level demands more.

The average person has 10 to 12 gallons of water in his or her body. To maintain this level, we need about three quarts of water a day under normal conditions. Fresh fruits, vegetables, and food may provide about half. (Fruits and vegetables are more than 90 percent water. Even dry foods contain water—bread is 35 percent and crackers are 5 percent water.) Water and beverages supply the rest.

To make water more interesting, squeeze a little lemon, lime, or mandarin orange into your glass.

A good idea is to keep a bottle or jug of water at hand and finish it by the end of the day. Try to drink water from glass containers. Soft plastic containers may possibly shed chemicals into the water (especially distilled water) and these may act as "hormone disruptors" to the immune and reproductive systems. It is conceivable, for example, that trucks carrying water in plastic containers could be detained in hot areas, overheating the inside of the trucks, leading to toxic

A great way to start each day to keep your body running smoothly is to drink two glasses of quality filtered water with one gram of vitamin C and an antioxidant. Finish the day with a glass of water. Optional: Add several capsules of herbs, such as echinacea, during the cold season, milk thistle several times a year for cleaning out your liver (or when you have eaten or drunk too much or had chemical exposures), or astragalus if you are fighting off an infection.

chemical exposure in the bottled water. Until more is known, it is probably better to purchase water in glass containers when possible, or in the hardest plastics (as the questionable compounds are used to make plastics soft and flexible). Another option is to buy a quality water filter for your home.

Why Not Water from the Tap?

The water that comes out of your tap is far from perfect. Household water starts from natural sources and goes through a number of cleaning treatments at the city water plants, which makes you assume that the water is now "perfectly safe." Wrong. The water that comes out of your faucet may contain harmful elements, such as synthetic compounds like fossil fuel emissions, industrial effluents, human wastes, detergents, and solvents that originate from contaminated sources; estrogenic chemicals; and agricultural runoff containing pesticides and fertilizers. Some of these are immune-depressing and cancer-promoting chemicals.

Metals, radionucleotides (which cause cancer), bacteria (such as cryptosporidium, a common contaminate that is immune to the action of chlorine), and viruses can make it through many treatment plants. For economic reasons, many problem substances are not filtered out by city water-treatment centers. Anything you take in through water will eventually circulate throughout all the tissues of your body. If your water comes from a private well, have it tested every several years.

General Intestinal Exercises and Reflex Points

Do the following simple exercises several times a week for a month, or whenever your digestion is "off." If you have severe digestive problems, do them several times a day for the first week and once a day for the second.

Exercises

- *Stomach Flapping.* Stand up with your hands on your knees. Lean over slightly. Inhale. Exhale fully. With your breath held out, pull your stomach in as far as it will go, then suddenly release it all the way out—"flap it out." Do this back and forth ten times on one exhale. Repeat three times.
- *Abdominal Roll.* Stand up. Roll abdomen and pelvis around in circles, first to the right, then to the left. Do 10 circles to the right, then 10 circles to be left. While you are moving, with lightly closed fists *gently* percuss, or lightly tap, your abdomen. (Your body sends energy to where you percuss.)
- *Intestinal Hand Massage.* Lie down and relax. Think of your favorite place. Pretend you are there. With the three middle fingers of each hand, gently massage your abdomen in little circles. Massage up your right side, across the top beneath your ribs, and down the left side to your pubic bone. If you

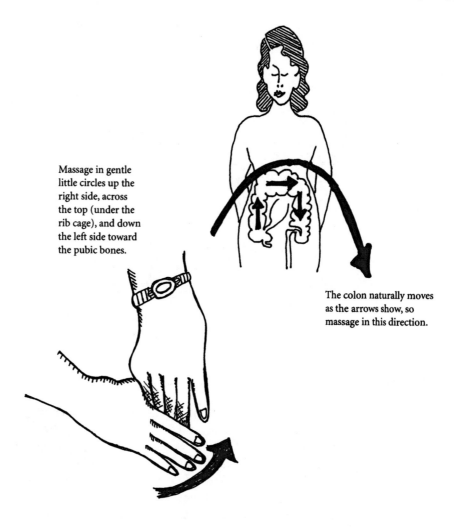

Massage in gentle little circles up the right side, across the top (under the rib cage), and down the left side toward the pubic bones.

The colon naturally moves as the arrows show, so massage in this direction.

feel any tension, tightness, or pain, work it out (gently rub until you feel the tension relax). Take a moment to inhale into the area and imagine that your healing breath is relaxing this area.

- *General Digestive Reflex Treatment.* Rub digestive areas on your feet with your thumb or knuckle. If you find a tender spot or feel a gritty nodule, give it special time and attention. While you are working this area, gently breathe into your abdomen. Work out all the tender spots on the whole digestive tract (stomach, intestines, colon, and anus)—go up the right foot from the heel to the middle, across to the instep, across the left foot instep to the outside and down to the heel—until they are perceptibly less sore or not tender at all.

To finish, hold the center of each foot with your thumbs while taking a few deep breaths to relax.

3 *Intestinal Protectors*

If you frequently eat doughnuts for breakfast, hamburgers for lunch, and steak for dinner, without fresh fruits and vegetables or high-fiber foods, your colonic environment is most probably *out of balance*.

If you live under chronic stress or have taken several courses of antibiotics for infections over the last several years and haven't used friendly bacteria to "re-seed" your colon, your intestinal protectors are probably lying down on the job.

Understanding Your Intestinal Ecology

We hear much these days about the importance of global ecology. This new vision of the earth as one huge interrelated ecosystem, where each country's pollution affects that of every other country, is at the core of our understanding that everything affects everything else.

This interconnectedness holds true within our bodies. Your body is an interrelated ecosystem in which *everything affects everything else.* One important component of this ecosystem is the intestinal environment. *Half* of all the material within your intestines are microbes (minute living organisms). Together they weigh from 3 to 4 pounds, similar in size to a single kidney. There are *friendly* organisms (protectors, called *probiotics*) and potentially *harmful* organisms (invaders, called *pathogens*) inside your intestinal tract, predominately in the large intestine (the colon). Balance or imbalance between these kinds of organisms can have wide-reaching effects on the quality of your health.

There are more cells of friendly bacteria inside your body than there are cells that make up your entire body. Friendly bacteria live in, on, and around the intestinal lining like a healthy green lawn. The healthier a lawn is, the less it can be invaded by unwanted weeds, whereas weeds easily take root and grow in an unhealthy lawn. In a similar way, friendly bacteria protect against a wide variety of unfriendly bacteria.

Vaginal births help to set the stage for optimal intestinal flora. Gut flora in infants born by *Caesarian* delivery are disturbed for up to six months or more. Normal intestinal flora is a prerequisite for intestinal immunity, which is imperative to ward off allergies, infections, and cancer.

Not Enough Friendly Bacteria

Because of disruptive factors in our external and internal environments, this optimal balance between friendly and unfriendly organisms in the intestinal tract may be adversely altered, if not reversed. Such an altered or unhealthy balance is called intestinal *dysbiosis*.

Bacterial tests on fecal samples show that many of us are walking around with greatly reduced friendly bacteria.

There are many possible causes for the imbalance between friendly and unfriendly bacteria: a diet high in stressor foods (junk food diet); life stress; steroid drugs (including cortisone, prednisone, and birth control pills); repeated exposure to antibiotics, both directly from prescriptions and indirectly from animal foods (antibiotics are given to animals to avoid infection); decreased or increased intestinal transit time (diarrhea or constipation); and intestinal parasites or fungal infections.

CHRONIC STOMACHACHES AND VAGINAL INFECTIONS

Jane was an active housewife and mom, but she was having trouble. Several hours after lunch, every day like clockwork, she'd get a stomachache, and once a month she'd get a vaginal yeast infection with plenty of irritation and itching.

She tried suppositories, cotton panties, eating more fiber, and eating less fruit, but nothing helped. Finally, Jane ended up at my clinic. I told her about the benefits of friendly bacteria found in yogurt. She started to eat one cup of yogurt twice daily. In a short time her stomachaches and vaginal problem left and, as a bonus, her skin cleared up. Jane was amazed that the answer to her problems could be so simple.

How Friendly Bacteria Protect Us

Friendly bacteria (probiotics) include *L. acidophilus, L. bulgaris, L. casei, L. bifidus, L. salivarius, streptococcus lactis,* and *streptococcus thermophilus,* to mention a few. They can:

- *Make Short-Chain Fatty Acids.* Probiotics break down carbohydrates in the large intestine into short-chain fatty acids (SCFAs), which supply both the intestinal tract and the body with energy. SCFAs are essential for a healthy colon and for maintaining healthy intestinal barrier functions.
- *Assist Digestion and Digestive Disorders.* Friendly bacteria produce some digestive enzymes. They have been used to improve maldigestion and to aid digestive disorders such as constipation and diarrhea, as well as indigestion,

How do you know if you have enough friendly bacteria in your intestines? Microscopic analysis of your stool measures certain factors that indicate the balance of your intestinal ecology. Ask your holistic doctor (See appendix B).

belching, and gas. Friendly bacteria appear to increase absorption of minerals, such as calcium, magnesium, and sometimes iron. These organisms have been used to improve intestinal disorders, such as peptic ulcer, irritable bowel syndrome, colitis, and inflammatory bowel disease.

- *Act like Natural Antibiotics.* A number of friendly bacteria can produce natural protective products—antibacterial, antifungal, and antiviral substances. This means these substances inhibit or kill disease-causing bacteria, fungi, or viruses. Thus, friendly bacteria indirectly protect the immune system.
- *Maintain Optimal Intestinal pH.* Friendly bacteria help maintain a proper intestinal pH (acid-alkaline balance), which optimizes digestion and further protects against disease-causing organisms that grow in abnormally altered pHs.
- *Help Digest Fats.* Friendly bacteria digest fats into healthy fatty acids, and help lower cholesterol.
- *Make B Vitamins.* Friendly bacteria make certain B vitamins (biotin, niacin, folic acid, pantothenic acid, vitamin B_{12}, and vitamin B_6).
- *Protect Against Cancer.* Friendly bacteria directly or indirectly help produce a variety of by-products (such as lignins) that protect against certain cancers and other disease-causing substances.
- *Assist Detoxification.* Friendly bacteria detoxify bile in the intestinal tract and deactivate many toxic pollutants.
- *Protect Women.* Some friendly bacteria indirectly contribute to optimal estrogen balance within the female body. Excessive exposure to estrogen is thought to be associated with a wide range of female health problems, from severe PMS to certain cancers.
- *Protect Against Parasites.* Friendly bacteria keep some parasites from transforming into more aggressive, disease-causing strains. Studies have shown that if bacterial flora from a person infected with *aggressive* amoebae are mixed with *unaggressive* amoebae, the unaggressive amoebae can "transform" into an aggressive strain. The reverse is also true.
- *Protect Against Food Allergies.* Friendly bacteria help maintain an optimal intestinal lining, which protects against allergy-causing substances.

How to Get Friendly Bacteria

Eat cultured products such as yogurt, kefir, milk, and cottage cheese. The label should state the product contains live cultures. Creative and easy ways to consume these products are offered later in this chapter.

Eat a diet high in whole grains, vegetables, and fruits. These "good foods" feed "good bacteria." Avoid stressor foods, such as fatty foods and refined sugars, as these adversely alter the intestinal environment, making it difficult for friendly bacteria to thrive (see chapter 1).

Be encouraged! Recent studies show that altering and improving your diet or bowel transit time can improve your friendly flora within a few weeks.

The B vitamins, especially vitamin B$_1$, folic acid, and pantothenic acid, contribute to an intestinal environment that promotes friendly bacteria. Taking vitamin C along with the B vitamins may potentiate this action.

Use raw apple-cider vinegar as an ingredient in your salad dressing, or sip it in water with a little raw honey as a beverage to promote the growth of friendly bacteria. Use it along with olive oil over steamed vegetables for flavor and health.

Nutritional yeast (*Saccharomyces cerevisiae*) is a potent source of protein, vitamins, minerals, and acts like a *probiotic*. Avoid if you have Crohn's disease or difficulties handling yeast. Its glucose tolerance factor is helpful for lowering blood sugar in diabetics. Add probiotics slowly to your diet. If you add too much too soon, you can get gas or irritation for a short period of time.

The Most Famous Friendly Bacteria

My favorite cultured food dish is a mix of blueberries, a little applesauce, ground flaxseeds, and some raw rolled oats or rye with nonfat organic yogurt. I stir and let it sit in the fridge for at least an hour, and then enjoy it by the spoonful. It tastes like cheesecake.

Lactobacillus acidophilus is almost a household word, since it has become commercially available in dairy products (yogurt, *acidophilus* milk, and kefir) as well as in *lactobacillus* powders and tablets. But what exactly is it? The name *Lactobacillus* can be confusing because there are numerous species of it, of which *L. acidophilus* is only one. *L. acidophilus* is a natural inhabitant of the human small intestine, the mouth, and the vagina.

L. acidophilus produces the enzyme *lactase*, which helps digest *lactose*, a milk sugar. Milk-intolerant people lack lactase and therefore cannot digest milk products. These folks often experience abdominal discomfort, gas, and bloating after consuming cow's-milk products. On the other hand, *cultured* cow's-milk products make milk sugar, and even milk proteins, easier to digest. This means that yogurt and kefir, which contain live cultures of *L. acidophilus*, can be enjoyed by many (but not all) milk-intolerant people.

L. acidophilus has a number of unique actions:

It promotes a healthy acid-alkaline balance, which inhibits the overgrowth of unfriendly bacteria. Lactobacillus is so effective in this manner that it has been given to elderly patients after surgery to avoid massive bacterial overgrowth that can cause blood poisoning.

It improves immune-system function. It inhibits overgrowth of "hostile" yeasts, such as *Candida albicans,* and reduces the manufacture of cancer-causing chemicals in the intestinal tract, thus possibly helping prevent colon cancer. One study of a strain of lactobacilli (*L. casei*) has shown it to decrease recurrences of bladder cancer and another has been shown to reduce cavities.

Promotes optimal cholesterol levels and reduces the risk of heart disease. Consuming one cultured product a day containing *L. acidophilus* has been shown to reduce cholesterol levels from 2.4 to 4 percent in less than a month, which is thought to help reduce the risk of heart disease by 6 to 10 percent. Studies of the effects of *L. acidophilus* on healthy folks, from African Masai warriors to bottle-fed babies, suggest that eating fermented milk products that contain live cultures promotes optimal cholesterol levels.

There are conflicting opinions about the success of these organisms in treating vaginitis in women. Some studies show they are effective in treating and preventing relapse of vaginitis, whereas others suggest that intravaginal application of yogurt for treating vaginitis is rarely effective. One reason for this discrepancy may be that what you get is not necessarily what the label advertised.

Yogurt Can Be More Effective Than Drugs

Forty patients with cirrhosis (severe liver disease) were randomly separated into two groups. One group was given friendly bacteria (two cups of yogurt three times a day) and the other group was treated with customary medication. The lactobacillus bacteria were shown to be as effective as drugs in lowering blood ammonia levels, and the people receiving the yogurt had no toxic side effects and felt better in general. The beneficial results lasted longer than those of the drugs.

L. sporogenes is another friendly strain that survives the acid in the stomach. It appears to be more stable than *L. acidophilus*, yet offers many similar benefits. Unlike *L. acidophilus*, it doesn't require refrigeration, so this probiotic is a good one to take along when you travel.

Yogurt and Kefir—Two Strong Allies

Balkan communities used to pass down "starter" cultures of yogurts from one generation to another. The making of cultured products was cherished as a culinary and medicinal "art." Cultured foods contain many nutrients in easily assimilated forms. They are higher in protein than milk. The milk proteins and sugars are in a more digestible form than those found in milk. The milk proteins in yogurt are fermented into digestible substances that healthfully stimulate the liver, enhance digestion, and inhibit the growth of unfriendly bacteria.

Add yogurt and kefir to your diet. Try rice, soy, or goat milks, which contain added cultured products. Learn to enjoy different flavors and at the same time enhance your health.

According to a 1990 study, out of sixteen *L. acidophilus* products from local pharmacies, grocery stores, and health-food stores, *only four contained L. acidophilus*. One product contained bacterial contaminants. What does this mean to you? *Buy only from reputable companies. And try to puchase products containing several strains of lactobacillus.*

Creative Ways to Eat Yogurt

- Mix yogurt with applesauce or shredded apples and raisins.
- Spread yogurt on toast with apple butter on top.
- Mix yogurt with diced cucumbers, tomatoes, and onions and serve on toasted bagel.

- Mix yogurt with hot whole-grain cereal and one teaspoon of sugarless organic fruit spread, and stir well.
- Mix yogurt with carob chips and trail mix, or granola.
- Mix yogurt with ground flaxseeds and cut-up fresh fruit, or one teaspoon of sugarless fruit spread or applesauce. Optional: Try appleberry sauce.

Bifidobacteria

These bacteria—a cousin to Lactobacilla—are the predominate friendly bacteria found in breast-fed infants. Bifidobacteria "infantus" used to make up almost 100 percent of the microflora in the intestines of breast-fed babies. However, studies show that today's babies, even breast-fed ones, have less Bifidobacteria. As soon as babies start to eat solid food, their microflora starts to look like that of adults—now containing lactobacillus, along with other friendly probiotics and, to a lesser degree, Bifidobacteria.

These organisms also protect your stomach from the possible adverse side effects of some food additives. Many processed meats—hot dogs, salami, sausage, even some turkey—have sodium nitrite added to preserve color and to destroy the bacteria that cause food poisoning. Nitrites are converted within the intestines into harmful nitrosamines, which are associated with an increased risk of stomach cancer. *L. acidophilus*, Bifidobacteria, and vitamin C block production of nitrosamines.

You may think that by buying turkey you are doing something healthy. Read the label. You'll find that most commercial brands contain nitrites, even at deli counters where the meat is sliced to order. Ask for nitrite-free meats or shop at a health-food store that carries nitrite- and antibiotic-free meats.

Protective Eating Hints

- If you have sausage for breakfast, take a little vitamin C (several hundred mgs)
- If you eat a hot dog, have yogurt for dessert.
- If you eat a bologna sandwich, drink some kefir as a beverage.
- If you make a sandwich from processed turkey, use yogurt instead of mayonnaise. If this tastes too bland, mix it with mustard and/or horseradish.

Taking Probiotics Wisely

Bifidobacteria and *L. acidophilus* appear to work together to protect against the growth of harmful organisms, enhance liver metabolism, and produce B vitamins. As a dietary supplement, the dose for both organisms to be effective is 1 to 10 billion viable organisms a day—equal to several capsules two to four times a day.

Lactobacilli are destroyed by moisture, sunlight, and heat. Heat is generated in making tablets. Thus lactobacilli should be freeze-dried, in powder or capsules, in opaque containers. Most *L. acidophilus*, except spore-forming strains, require refrigeration and should be in a cooler at the store and refrigerated at home. Labels should state that the product contains live cultures (unless the product is spore-forming) and give a specific expiration date.

You will notice that some products contain FOS. FOS stands for *fructo-oligosaccharides*, large vegetable fiber and complex sugars. It is a food for the organisms to live on and encourages the growth of Bifidobacteria, while restricting the growth of potential pathogens. FOS is concentrated in garlic, onion, asparagus, artichokes, and chicory root, and may be produced synthetically.

These products are best taken with meals.

More Easy Ways to Get Friendly Bacteria

- Eat cultured vegetables, such as raw sauerkraut (available at health-food stores) or dilly beans. Sauerkraut contains *L. plantarum*, which remains in the intestine long after being eaten.
- Eat cottage cheese with added probiotics.
- Make morning smoothies with kefir or yogurt. Add protein powder, fruit, and water, then blend.

Therapeutic Uses for Friendly Bacteria

Researchers at Harvard have shown that Bifidobacteria, along with FOS, helps heal defects in the intestinal lining and labels their use as *eco-immune nutrition*.

Consider adding probiotics to your treatment "bag" for constipation, ulcers, hemorrhoids, gallstones, irritable bowel syndrome, colitis, inflammatory bowel disease, or any general intestinal discomfort. Probiotics have been shown to be helpful for diarrhea caused by infection, antibiotics, traveling, and even for recurrent diarrhea caused by treatment for *Clostridium difficile* infection.

- Take 2 to 3 capsules for diarrhea, constipation, or heartburn two to three times a day for several weeks, or at least two weeks after the symptoms go away.
- Take 3 to 4 capsules three to four times a day after a round of antibiotics, for two weeks to one month.
- Take 2 to 3 capsules two to three times a day after any type of major surgery, for one to two weeks.

- Take 3 to 4 capsules three to four times a day after food poisoning, for two or three days.
- Consume a bowl of yogurt a day to *prevent* diarrhea while traveling abroad. Consume several bowls of yogurt a day to *treat* traveler's diarrhea.
- If you have food allergies, strains of lactobacillus can reduce some food hypersensitivities and protect the barrier function of the gut.
- *Saccharomyces boulardii* has been used for years in Europe to treat acute diarrhea and to prevent antibiotic-induced diarrhea (one case of adverse fungal infection with it has been reported).
- *Lactobacillus salivarius* looks like a promising new treatment for *H. pylori,* a bug that can cause ulcers and is associated with gastritis and stomach cancer (but these new studies have been in test tubes, not yet in humans).

Note: *Severely* immune-suppressed people with impaired gut barrier should not use probiotics, as these live organisms may cross the lining and be absorbed.

4 *Using Your Mind-Body Link to Maximize Digestive Wellness*

Scientists are discovering that we are indeed a complex web of interconnectedness, in which many of our parts—and our minds and bodies—influence and affect each other.

Is the Mind-Body Link Real?

At a Medicine and Spirituality conference sponsored by Harvard Medical School in 1997, the body-mind connection was discussed before an audience of 1,500 doctors and associated clergy. Dr. Herbert Benson opened the conference by stating that "the mind and body are one unit and that it was science, not spirituality, that led to this convergence." Three decades of research at Harvard's Mind/Body Institute had convinced Dr. Benson that health and well-being require not only pharmaceuticals, medical care, and surgery, but also *self-care*—a combination of mind-body issues, paying attention to nutrition, exercise, meditation, and spirituality. Dr. Benson defined spirituality as a striving for emotional peace, relaxation, and a sense of connection to some kind of healing power.

Some studies exploring this mind-body link emphasize another factor—the intestinal tract. The intestinal tract, brain, and immune systems greatly influence and communicate with each other through specific proteins. This has been dubbed the "brain-immune-gut axis." Many of the investigations of this axis explore the effects that imagery, meditation, affirmation, relaxation, and biofeedback have on these systems.

Your Brain and Your Gut

You learned in chapter 1 that the intestinal tract has such a huge system of nerves, comparable to the number in the spinal cord, that it is said to have its

On the molecular level, you have no secrets. You aren't just what you digest, you are also what you think.

own brain, and that 80 percent of your immune system lines the intestinal tract. You may also remember that the intestinal tract has the largest blood supply in the body. Researchers are now also discovering that receptors for hormones are found all along the length of the intestinal tract.

Why in the world would your intestinal tract have so much contact and communication with your immune, hormonal, nervous, and blood systems? Because these are all the signaling systems in your body that communicate the messages of life, that dictate to all your cells what to do and inform them about what is going on. This intricate network makes your intestinal tract instantaneously responsive to your thoughts and emotions, not just to your diet and nutrients. When your emotions are set into gear, they affect these systems, which mutually connect and affect your mind and your immune and digestive capabilities.

In my opinion, it is here, at the lining of your intestinal tract, that the two essential facets of nourishment intersect—nutrients and thoughts. I believe that thoughts and nutrients are the two most important foods for your mind and body. As simple as this sounds, I believe you need to eat the best food and think the best thoughts in order to maintain harmony and wholeness of body and mind. How you think affects how you assimilate food. How you assimilate food affects how you think.

A TALE OF ULCERS AND MEDITATION

Lisa, a single mom in her early twenties, had a full-time job as a receptionist at a surgeon's office. She got an ulcer, which medication healed at first, but even on maintenance medication, the ulcer kept recurring. Lisa was exhausted and tired of hurting.

She heard about a yoga teacher who worked with health problems. She enrolled in a class and began to meditate. The teacher taught Lisa imagery, meditation, and affirmation techniques. With nothing other than her own efforts to quiet her mind and use her innate healing energies, Lisa had no more recurrences. Now, from personal experience, she enthusiastically recommends meditation to many of the surgery patients who come into her workplace.

Explanation of Terms

What is *imagery*? Imagery is creating an internal experience without actually living it in the external environment. Imagery is using imagination, or what is called "visualization," to attempt to influence reality.

Dr. Stephen Kosslyn, professor of psychology at Harvard University, has demonstrated that imagery activates the same areas of the brain that are activated when we actually see something in front of us in physical reality. About 65 percent of the areas of the brain used in vision are used in imagery. In other words, when you imagine or visualize something, the brain acts exactly as if you were actually looking at it.

Thus, imagery acts like perception. These perceptions can modify how people handle pain and how fast they heal.

According to Dr. Kosslyn, "imagery is not mystical or unstructurable and it is amenable to science." More research needs to be done, but according to experts like Dr. Kosslyn, "imagery could be utilized to help one change the hormonal and immunological state of one's body."

What are *affirmations?* Affirmations are positive mental "statements," or verbal mental imagery that you repeat over and over to "train" your thoughts to influence your body. Affirmations are exercises to *flex* thought power.

Relaxation is created by deep breathing, body awareness, release of tension, and meditation.

Meditation is an exercise to quiet the mind, similar to thought-stopping techniques used in different forms of psychotherapies.

Proving the Mind-Body Link

One of the larger areas of research in mind-body medicine has been the intestinal tract. Learning to focus attention on your intestinal tract, while relaxing your body and mind, has been shown to assist healing. Dr. Jeanne Achterberg and associates measured an immune factor that lines the intestinal tract before and after imagery training, with and without music. She and her colleagues found that imagery and music significantly increased antibody production. At the same time, the patients felt better and had fewer symptoms.

Imagery can influence and perhaps optimize physiological functioning within body cells, including the intestinal tract. In a unique study at Michigan State University, subjects using imagery were able to *train* white blood cells to perform feats not normally performed by white blood cells.

Recent advances in the investigation of the brain-gut "cross-talk" suggest that the role of the brain is influential in intestinal diseases. In the eighties, Dr. Candice Pert isolated an intestinal protein that had communication sites in the brain as well as in immune tissue. Other proteins have since been found to have communication (receptor) sites on the intestinal tract. This all points to an exciting, complex web of interconnectedness between your intestinal tract, brain, nervous system, and immune system.

Cross-talk within the intestinal tract also occurs between cells involved in allergic response and nerve fibers, both being close communicating neighbors. Researchers from the Institute of Internal Medicine in Rome believe that the closeness of these neighboring cells accounts for the nervous system (mood) directly influencing the intestinal tract and vice versa. They suggest this is one reason that anxiety, depression, food allergies, and bowel complaints (such as irritable bowel syndrome) often occur together in the same patient.

A number of studies use relaxation and meditation to treat intestinal disorders such as irritable bowel syndrome and ulcers. The Orlando General Hospital translated studies like these into techniques for people with many health problems, from intestinal complaints such as irritable bowel syndrome to immune problems like cancer. The authors said that imagery was the essential "backbone" of their program.

Studies reveal that guided imagery makes abdominal surgery less painful, which lessens the need for pain medication, decreases anxiety and stress, and increases sensations of well-being. Women who went through hysterectomies while listening to tapes of positive suggestions needed less pain medication and had less anxiety than other women. A study presented at the American Society of Colon and Rectal Surgeons in 1996 showed that guided imagery significantly reduced anxiety and pain after surgery to the lower colon.

Now the physiological effectiveness of both affirmations and prayer are being investigated. Two studies on long-distance healing, both scientifically controlled and randomized (hallmarks of scientific design), demonstrated significant health improvements with affirmation and prayer. One famous study was done by Dr. Rand Byrd (1988) on 393 cardiac patients at the coronary unit of San Francisco General Hospital. Dr. Byrd randomly assigned a prayer group to pray for some of his patients, while others were not prayed for. The "prayed for" patients had fewer complications and left the hospital earlier.

A second study by R. N. Miller (1982) had eight healers from the Church of Religious Science do remote healing on half of 96 patients suffering from high blood pressure. Neither the doctors nor the patients knew who received the remote healing. The healers relaxed, attuned with a higher power, visualized, and affirmed the patient to be in a perfect state of health, and ended with an expression of thanks. "Treatment"—in other words, this type of remote healing—continued for several weeks. Blood pressure was significantly reduced in the treated group. In fact, three healers had a perfect score—100 percent of their patients improved, compared with 73.9 percent in the control group.

According to Dr. Stephen M. Kosslyn, imagery is the most effective technique of all to manage pain. During his talk at the Medicine and Spirituality Conference, on neurobiological mechanisms related to the placebo effect, Dr. Kosslyn said: "Every study on imagery but one demonstrates a positive effect on reducing pain. This especially relates to pain that comprises stabbing, burning and pressing sensations." Because the types of pain described by Dr. Kosslyn are the most common types of pains associated with many gastrointestinal problems, these particular tools of healing are suggested for most of the conditions in this book.

You can use relaxation, meditation, and imagery to enhance healing, or you can skip these sections and focus on nutrition and exercise.

How to Use the Mind-Body Response

I interpret studies like the ones mentioned above to suggest that your gut, brain, and immune systems constantly talk to each other. Affirmations, imagery, and meditation, I believe, allow you to get in on these conversations.

According to experts like Dr. Herbert Benson, there are essential steps to creating effective healing through meditation, imagery, and relaxation.

Essential Steps to Healing through Meditation

- Expect that what you do *will work*. In other words, *expect to get well*.
- While sitting or lying down, tighten all your muscles as best you can for about 30 seconds, then LET GO and start to *relax*.
- Do this by slow, deep *breathing* and conscious relaxation of each body part (start at one end and work through your entire body), putting mind and body in a receptive state.
- *Meditate* on some words (they can be anything from saying that you are healing this part of your body to even just saying a simple word like "thanks" or "peace" or a mantra—spiritual words) that you repeat over and over while keeping a relaxed state of being. Benson's research suggests that repeating one word may be more effective than using multiple words.
- *Visualize* that you are well, that this part of your body is healing.
- Finish by *affirming* that you are being healed or give thanks for being healed (whichever appeals most to your world-life point of view).

At the end of most chapters in this book are simple breathing techniques, meditations, visualizations, and affirmations—mind-body techniques to help you heal your health problems. Do each exercise once a day for one week. Experience how becoming more aware of your "center" influences your overall well-being. Then try the other exercises offered at the end of most of the chapters. These types of exercises improve digestion and overall health, as well as make you more aware of how you *live* inside your body. Specific words for affirmations are suggested, but you can substitute your own.

The following exercises are excellent to do when embarking on healing any type of digestive problem.

Meditation for Intestinal Awareness

Put on gentle music or be in a quiet room. Burn a candle or let a gentle breeze blow across you. Lie comfortably with your arms by your sides, palms facing the ceiling. Bend your knees and place your feet by your buttocks so your back is relaxed.

Take three deep breaths. Then take your awareness to your abdomen. How does your abdomen *feel*? What does this mean? Your abdomen is the *center* of your body. People who practice all the martial arts, yoga, and meditation forms, even dancers and athletes, realize that the center of the body's energy comes from this place near the belly button. This center of energy is referred to by many names, such as *Hara, t'an t'ien,* and *center of gravity.*

Be aware that this is your body's center of energy and that it influences all aspects of health. You can "feel" if your center is strong or weak, healthy or blocked. Over time, you not only become aware of how it feels, but you will be able to strengthen it. That is your goal, to develop communication with the center of your body and be able to strengthen it when it is weak.

Start by drawing your awareness to the area around your navel. Inhale. Fill your abdomen as much as you can, pushing your abdomen with the breath up toward the ceiling. As you exhale, hum out loud the sound "Hmmmm." As you hum, gently let your abdomen fall back toward the floor, toward your spine. Repeat for five to fifteen minutes, or whatever length of time is comfortable. Keep this up long enough to become filled with the sound, so that there is a sense of vibrating. Feel this vibration inside you. When you have had enough, stop.

Now, once again, as in the beginning, try to go within. Become aware of how your center feels. How does the length of your intestinal tract feel? Compare how your center feels now to how it felt when you first started this exercise.

This is self-exploration. Just as you know your face, you should *know* how your intestinal tract, your center, is *feeling*. Practice this meditation every night for one week. By the end of that week you will have a better understanding of what your center feels like and when it is tense or relaxed.

Affirmations for Intestinal Awareness and Healing

Sit or lie comfortably. Close your eyes. Bring your awareness to your breath. Inhale and exhale deeply three times. Start with your toes and tighten them. Then move up your body and tighten each part until your arms and legs and head are a little off the floor, very tight. Tighten a little more. Then, when tightened to the maximum, exhale and completely relax.

With each *inhale* say, "*Relax.*"

Remind your body to let go of tension.

With each *exhale* say, "*Completely.*"

Let this relaxation fill your body. After you feel more relaxed than when you started, take your awareness to your abdomen. Inhale as though you could direct your breath to your abdomen.

On the *inhale* say, "*I heal my digestion.*"

On the *exhale,* say, "*I relax my digestion.*"

Repeat for five to ten minutes. This develops the ability to know what it feels like to relax your intestinal tract. Once you know what it feels like to have a relaxed intestinal tract, you can use this during your day or in stressful situations.

For example, during the day you can focus your awareness on your intestines. If they feel "tense and tight," you can change this. Breathe in and out. "Tell" your intestines to relax. Get them to feel as they do during these intestinal meditations and affirmations. That's what meditations and affirmations are for. They should spill over into your life, positively influencing your daily habits.

PART II

Specific Digestive Conditions

Gas and Bloating
Heartburn
Constipation
Diarrhea
Diverticular Disease
Hemorrhoids
Inflammatory Bowel Disease
Peptic Ulcers
Gallbladder Disease
Irritable Bowel Syndrome
Other Causes of Intestinal Pain
Mouth and Gum Conditions
Intestinal Parasites
The Candida-Related Complex
Colorectal Cancer and AIDS

5 *Easy Ways to Get Rid of Gas and Bloating*

You don't have to suffer from abdominal bloating, discomfort, or embarrassing flatulence. There are simple home remedies to give you relief from either chronic (habitual and continual) or acute (sudden and severe) gas symptoms. But most important, these symptoms are often signals that you are not properly digesting your food.

Chapter 1 introduced the digestion triangle. The three major points on the triangle are food absorption, assimilation, and elimination. Chronic bloating, gas, belching, and abdominal discomfort are often early signals suggesting that this triad is being adversely affected.

Chronic excess gas is predominately made up of *methane*, which may deplete specific short-chain fatty acids (SCFAs) that are important food for the lining of the colon, leaving it more prone to premalignant polyps and cancer. Also, people with chronic excess gas, "methane formers," have more *sulfate-reducing bacteria* in their feces. These cause a higher level of sulfides in the feces, which is associated with more disease of the colon. Thus, you should understand that chronic gas is not just a drag, it's a risk factor for intestinal problems.

CHERYL'S MYSTERIOUS BACK PAIN

Cheryl was a young aspiring opera singer. She came to see me for chronic back pain that was threatening her career. The pain made it almost impossible for her to stand for long hours and sing. She had tried massage, exercise, chiropractic treatments, and extended physiotherapy. They had all failed to relieve the severe, constant pain that ran down the right side of her back and into her hip. Cheryl was surprised because I asked about her digestion. She didn't think digestion had anything to do with her back. I explained that her muscles were very sensitive to her nutritional status, especially her tissue levels of calcium and magnesium. I further explained that poor digestion of these minerals created a perfect environment for chronic muscle spasms.

It turned out that Cheryl suffered from chronic gas. After every meal she had to let out her belt, and often had to go to a bathroom to privately relieve herself of flatus (gas). We ran a test that measured the amount of stomach acid (hydrochloric acid) made in Cheryl's stomach and found that she produced inadequate levels. We treated her with stomach acid capsules, and in one week, Cheryl's three-year back pain problem ended. She was delighted to be able to stand and sing long arias without any pain. Cheryl's story demonstrates how digestive problems can be related to many other types of health concerns.

Ten Typical Symptoms of Gas

1. Distention: Pants or belt feel tighter after eating.
2. Fullness: Uncomfortably full after eating normal amounts of food.
3. Abdominal discomfort after eating.
4. Intermittent waves of pain or heightened discomfort.
5. Passing flatus to the point that it is bothersome to yourself and others.
6. Belching to the point that it is bothersome to yourself and others.
7. Heartburn.
8. Pain: Gas pain can occur in the abdominal area as well as in the chest area and down the arm (mimicking a heart attack), in the back, and sometimes at the level of the breast bone.
9. Coated tongue.
10. Nausea.

Common Causes of Gas

- Irritation to the lining of the gastrointestinal tract due to excessive consumption of caffeinated and alcoholic beverages, refined sugar, excess salt, and/or processed oils.
- Eating too much.
- Nutrient deficiencies.
- Digestive enzyme deficiencies.
- Food allergies or intolerances (not a true allergy but still causes a problem).
- Gallbladder dysfunction or inadequate bile.
- Sugar intolerances: Deficiencies in enzymes that digest sugars, such as milk sugars, and some fruit sugars, such as those found in apple and pear juice. (See chapter 14 for more details on sugar intolerances.)
- Emotional stress.
- Intestinal bacteria imbalance.
- Gases in foods (such as carbonated beverages).
- Candida-related complex (see chapter 16).

- Parasites.
- Other underlying health problems, such as problems with ovaries, fallopian tubes, or other pelvic organs.
- Air swallowed with food, or drinking too many carbonated or ice-cold beverages.

Abdominal flatulence, with pale, bad-smelling bowel movements and, possibly, unexplained weight loss, may be associated with malabsorption syndrome, parasites, bacterial imbalance, or in rare cases, a pancreatic tumor. See a professional.

Belching or gas that increases on bending over and lying down may signify a reflux of stomach acid in the esophagus (see chapter 6).

Gas associated with diarrhea and/or constipation, lower abdominal pain that lessens or goes away once gas is passed, and excessive gas accompanying most bowel movements may be indicative of intestinal problems such as colitis, irritable bowel syndrome, dysbiosis, parasites, or candida-related complex. See a doctor.

What to Do for *Chronic* Gas

Soothing Herbs

- Make a paste of honey, 1/2 teaspoon turmeric powder, and 1/2 teaspoon ginger powder. Mix and eat once a day for several weeks. Turmeric reduces the number of gas-forming bacteria.
- Put 1 teaspoon ginger powder or 2 tablespoons grated fresh ginger and 1/2 teaspoon fennel seeds per 1 cup of boiling water. Steep for five minutes. Sip during or after meal. Can drink hot or cold. Ginger contains about 400 active and beneficial ingredients.
- Add a pinch of cinnamon and clove to boiled water or tea and sip with meals.
- Try peppermint and/or licorice-root tea, well-steeped, 1 to 3 cups a day for two weeks.

Eight Food Tips

1. Chew slower.
2. Do not do anything else while eating.
3. Try eating only three food items per meal.
4. Try eating vegetables and fruits at separate meals.
5. Avoid eating melons at the end of a meal.
6. Stop eating refined sugars (or at least cut down).
7. Stop drinking fruit juices or colas with meals.
8. Eat less.

Supplements

Try two or three of the following for several *weeks:*

- *Pantothenic acid.* 1,000 to 2,000 mgs a day for the first week and then 500 mg once or twice a day. Pantothenic acid helps relieve intestinal gas and distention. *It is so effective it is recommended to postoperative patients with gas problems.*
- *B complex.* 50 mg of each once a day, with extra B_1 (25 mg) twice a day.
- *Aloe vera.* One tablespoon aloe vera juice in diluted fruit juice or water, twice a day between meals.

Other options:

- *Glutamine.* 500 mg one to three times a day for two months.
- *Hydrochloric acid* or *pancreatic enzymes.* As indicated, with meals (see chapter 19).

Food allergies should be identified and treated (see chapter 18).

What to Do for *Acute* Gas

Food Tips for Acute Gas, Bloating, and Belching

Don't eat any more food till your gas goes away and your abdomen feels better.
Sip hot tea made from fennel or peppermint, or both.
Sip hot water with the juice of a fresh lemon.
Sip hot water with 1 teaspoon of apple-cider vinegar and 1 tablespoon of honey.

Supplements for Acute Gas, Bloating, and Belching

Try one or two of the following items and see which works best for your body.

- Chew 3 to 4 chewable papaya enzymes or take 2 to 3 100-mg bromelain capsules.
- Try commercial "gas" formulas, available at your health-food store (see appendix B).
- Take 2 to 4 *L. acidophilus* capsules two to three times a day.
- Use digestive enzymes if indicated (see chapter 19).
- Take 2 activated charcoal tablets.

Charcoal is a strong absorbent agent. It has a lot of surface area to bind with undigested and toxic material to clear them out of the intestinal tract. Many water filters are made from charcoal because of this "cleansing" action. However, charcoal will bind up vital nutrients. Use it only for short periods of time until you figure out why you are having gas and bloat. Burned toast, in a pinch, has the same action.

Tips for Preventing Gas

Before eating, take a few breaths to quiet your body and mind to make your physiology more receptive to the food you are about to eat.

Eat a varied diet; avoid repeating the same foods every day. Avoid eating after 7 P.M. (The digestive tract is "winding down" later in the day. Night digestion is, in most people, less effective than digestion in the middle of the day.)

Emphasize: Fresh whole foods and cultured foods (label should state it contains *live* organisms).

Avoid: Fatty, spicy, and fried foods, overconsumption of red meats, meats with additives (nitrates), excessive consumption of refined sugars, alcoholic beverages, and sodas, coffee, and other caffeinated beverages. Especially avoid processed oils, hydrogenated oils, margarine, and rancid oils.

Optimal Juices for Less Gas

To prevent and treat chronic gas, consume one or two of any of the following juices each day for two to four weeks. You may blend the ingredients with water if you do not have a juicer, or if you want more natural fiber.

GI Morning Special   Juice several carrots, one Granny Smith apple, and one orange without the rind. Dilute with water.

GI Booster   Carrot, celery, with small slice of raw beet.

GI Tropical   Granny Smith apple, one carrot, fresh pineapple wedges, and several inches of fresh ginger.

Many years ago, I lived at the Hidden Valley Health Ranch in Escondido, California, studying with Dr. Bernard Jensen. He always praised the health benefits of greens. He devised a tasty green drink. Over the years I have created this variation:

Healing Green Drink   Stuff blender with a handful each of parsley and spinach, as well as four to five romaine lettuce leaves. Fill blender with pineapple juice or half juice and half water. Blend until mixture is smooth. Optional: Add mint leaves or raw seeds or nuts. Even though this is a "drink," be sure to chew well.

Remedies According to Patterns of Gas

WARNING: If your gas and bloating are accompanied by severe abdominal pains, sweating, paleness, or dizziness that persists for over six hours, see a doctor.

1. Gas and belching that occur **during, immediately after,** *or within a half hour of eating* suggests a stomach-acid deficiency or food allergy.

Try sipping 1 teaspoon organic apple-cider vinegar and 1 teaspoon honey in water.

Try sipping the juice of a fresh lemon in a glass of water throughout meal.

Take 1 to 3 betaine hydrochloride (8 to 10 grains) tablets with lactose-free pepsin, *throughout* the meal. (See chapter 19 to see if you need stomach acid, and how to take it.)

Identify your food allergies and eliminate these foods (see chapter 18).

2. Gas, belching, and bloating that occur *several hours after eating* suggest pancreatic enzyme deficiency, food allergies, and/or lactose (milk-sugar) intolerance.

Take 800 to 2,000 mg pancreatin after meals and/or identify possible food allergies and intolerances and avoid these foods. (A number of food allergies improve or go away once digestion is improved.) If you are also taking hydrochloric acid, take it during the meals and pancreatin after the meals.

Try eating less food types per meal.

3. Gas *within 1 to 1½ hours after eating* may suggest small-bowel overgrowth of unfriendly bacteria. (See chapter 20 to detoxify and rebuild, and read chapter 3 to understand intestinal ecology.)

4. Belching that worsens *after eating fatty foods*—possibly associated with sharp pain in upper right shoulder and/or abdomen and spreading to the back—may signify gallbladder disorder.

Eat less fatty foods, especially animal foods, such as cheese, red meat, and eggs. Especially avoid deep-fried foods, such as fries, fried chicken, fried zucchini strips, deep-fried potato skins, deep-fried corn chips, and onion rings.

Take bile acids (often come in multiple digestive enzyme formulas) and beet powder with meals for one to two months and explore the food allergy link. Consider hydrochloric acid capsules. (Read chapter 19 first; quite a number of gallbladder patients tend to be low in hydrochloric acid, and see chapter 13 on gallbladder functioning).

5. Gas and abdominal discomfort *with taking vitamin C.*

Cut down dosage of the vitamin C. When you start to slowly increase it again, add several hundred mg of bromelain several times a day for several days.

6. Gas, belching, and discomfort *after initiating new high-fiber diet, new vitamin regime, or increasing bean consumption.*

In my years as a nutritional consultant, many people came to me because they felt worse (gas, fatigue, nausea) when they had embarked on a new nutritional program. It wasn't the fault of the program, but that the person had started too much too soon.

When this happens:

Stop all new supplements.

Eat less high-fiber foods.

Drink extra water.

Take a little alkaline vitamin C (calcium ascorbate), two to three times a day on an empty stomach.

Wait to start anything new until all symptoms have stopped for several days. Add one new change per day. Then, go slowly to let your body acclimate. This also will allow you to identify what caused the problem.

Beans, Beans—the Magical Fruit

Beans have an eight-carbon ring sugar, raffinose, which is hard to digest. Many people do not have adequate stores of raffinase, the enzyme that breaks down this sugar. When undigested raffinose passes into the large intestine, it is fermented, acted on by bacteria, and causes gas.

Ways to Avoid a Gaseous Reaction When Eating Beans

Cooking: Soak beans for 8 hours in water with 1 tablespoon of ginger powder, or several pieces of fresh ginger. Discard water and then cook in new water with new ginger added. Or try cooking beans with several inches of a dried seaweed called *kombu*, which you can get at health-food stores.

Eat a smaller quantity of beans at one sitting.

Avoid eating beans with fatty foods, or cut down the amount of fatty foods. For example, ask for "light on the cheese" in Mexican restaurants.

Consume beans earlier in the day when digestion is most active.

Consume products with alpha-galactosidase, an enzyme from mold that helps digest beans (read labels to find which products contain this).

Mind-Body Techniques

Reflex Points for Gas

Press (for one minute in each location) the junction on the left hand where the thumb and the forefinger come together in a web. Then press in the center of the left hand. Feel for the most tender points in the center of the foot, especially under the ball of the left foot. Work the reflexes on the foot for the entire stomach, intestines, and rectal areas by rubbing with knuckles in small circles. Press and hold the most tender spots.

Easy Exercises for Gas

Breathing Exercise for Gas. Sit on heels on floor. If you cannot do this, then sit in a chair. Make fists with both hands. Place your fists into your abdomen. Put head on the ground, or if you are sitting, bend head on or near knees. Gently breathe deeply seven times. Then sit up and relax.

Intestinal Self-Massage. Lie on the floor by the side of your bed with your knees and feet on top of the bed. With your fingers, make small circular motions starting at your lower right side. Go up the right side of your abdomen, across your body (under your ribs), and down your left side toward your pubic bone. This is the path of your intestines. Repeat this pattern three times. Inhale and exhale three times. Relax for several minutes before getting up.

Do this massage once or twice a day for one to two weeks to improve overall intestinal health, intestinal transit time, and to reduce flatulence.

Affirmations

Sit comfortably. Take several deep breaths. Relax. Now, visualize breathing in cooling blue light with each inhalation. On the inhale, visualize this blue light filling up your intestines. On the exhale, visualize this blue light filling up your entire body.

Say to yourself on each inhale: *"I take in health."*

Say to yourself on each exhale: *"I let go of tension."*

Do this until your abdomen feels relaxed.

Repeat this once a day for one week and then several times a week for two to three more weeks.

6 *What to Do about Heartburn*

We often ignore the signals our bodies give us about a problem. Heartburn is an excellent example. Most people regard it as a nuisance, an "antacid deficiency." However, as you will learn, chronic heartburn is more commonly a signal that we have been abusing our diet or lifestyle.

The name heartburn is an umbrella term for common upper-abdominal discomfort described as "indigestion," fullness, gaseousness, abdominal distention, or gnawing and/or burning pain in the upper abdomen, chest, or behind the breastbone. It is common for heartburn to have a *burning* quality of pain, which gives it its name. Mild heartburn is annoying, but severe heartburn can be scary, feeling as if a hole were being burned through your stomach. Thus, it is easy to understand why people who suffer from this pain often resort to taking, if not living on, antacids.

Heartburn can exist by itself, or it can be a symptom of a disorder somewhere else in the digestive tract or body. To get rid of heartburn once and for all, you need to know what is causing it.

BOWLING AND HEARTBURN

Kirsten loved to bowl, but she had a problem. When she bent over to throw the bowling ball, a severe episode of heartburn would begin. She was living on antacids. The more antacids she took, the less energy she seemed to have.

I had Kirsten fill out a diet diary. It became apparent that Kristen didn't eat much throughout the day, but then ate a large meal with her family at night—and before she went out bowling. I recommended that Kirsten eat several small meals throughout the day. Just this reduction in eating allowed Kristen to strike it right at the bowling alley.

Common Causes of Heartburn

The following causes of heartburn emphasize how it is often the simple things we do or don't do that make the difference.

- *Overeating.* Too much food can cause pressure changes in your stomach, which push the stomach contents back up into the lower part of the esophagus. Even a moderate amount of food eaten late at night or after exercising may be interpreted by your body as "too much." Being overweight, pregnant, or wearing too-tight garments can also cause heartburn by exerting pressure upward on the stomach.
- *Eating too fast.* Chomping down on burgers or tacos in the car in traffic while rushing to your job? Insufficient chewing creates large pieces of food difficult for digestive enzymes to handle. This can cause heartburn.
- *Drinking too many caffeinated beverages, such as coffee, tea, or colas.* Chocolate abuse may also create heartburn because it contains caffeine and theobromine, another caffeinated substance.
- *Overeating refined carbohydrates,* such as sugars, breads, and pastas, especially accompanied by a low nutrient-fiber diet. Drinking two or more beers or glasses of wine at night may be causing your heartburn.
- *Smoking* can cause heartburn. This effect is exaggerated by smoking before or during a meal.

Gastroesophageal Reflux

You have a sphincter (valve) between your esophagus and stomach that is supposed to prevent your stomach contents from backing up into the more delicate lining of the esophagus. When this happens it is called *gastroesophageal reflux,* which causes heartburn.

Other factors can also cause this reflux: overeating; excessive consumption of acidic foods, such as tomato-based foods; a poor-functioning valve (sphincter); hiatal hernia; pregnancy (see later in this chapter); ulcers; disease or irritation of the esophagus; loss of intestinal-lining-protective factors that may be secondary to low stomach acid (see chapter 1); and inadequate nutrients, such as folic acid and vitamin A.

- Try eating fewer tomatoes and citrus fruits, and consuming less alcoholic beverages, especially red wine.
- Don't eat late at night.
- Don't drink late at night.
- Don't overconsume fluids with meals.

- Don't smoke.
- Eat less refined sugars, such as chocolates.

Specific Foods That Aggravate Gastroesophageal Reflux

Coffee, tea, cola, peppermint and spearmint (volatile oils called carminatives, which are often added to after-dinner liqueurs), onions, peppers, tomatoes and tomato-based sauces and foods, citrus, and fatty foods (especially animal fats and chocolate) may cause pressure changes in the stomach of sensitive people that can cause reflux and heartburn. Orange juice, in sensitive people, has been shown to disrupt normal muscular action of the lower portion of the esophagus.

Cut out these foods for a month. Reintroduce one food a day and see how you feel. Add them back sparingly into your diet if they do not cause an immediate problem. Avoid them completely if they do.

Other Causes of Heartburn

I found heartburn to be a common symptom in individuals who were tested and proven to produce too little stomach acid. However, it can be dangerous to take stomach acid if you are actually making too much of it (see chapter 19 for details).

Drugs can cause heartburn (hormones such as those in the birth control pill, and progesterone, diazepam, and nitroglycerine). Too much magnesium may cause heartburn in some people, as it is a natural muscle relaxant and the valve is a muscle of sorts.

Food allergies. According to Dr. James Breneman, past president of the American College of Allergists, persistent heartburn from a particular food is a reliable symptom of allergy to that food. He states that addiction to antacids is a common finding in the medical history of food-allergy patients. Food allergies stimulate histamine release, which stimulates stomach-acid secretion. Most common offenders are cow's-milk products, wheat, eggs, corn, beef, soy, and some citrus fruits.

Infection by a bug called *H. pylori.* Get a blood test (see chapter 12 on treatment).

Swallowing air during meals.

Stomach acid: too much or too little. Severe emotional stress can promote increased stomach acid secretion. This is caused by release of stress-related hormones during the stressful period, or even well after the stress has ended. Sometimes health problems related to stress, such as heartburn, may show up any time within two years of the stressful event.

Making insufficient levels of stomach acid can also cause heartburn. There are studies demonstrating that even people who suffer from achlorhydria, meaning they make little or no stomach acid, can experience heartburn. One study followed people who were low in stomach acid for ten years and about half of them complained of chronic heartburn.

Insufficient stomach acid creates indigestion and gas in the stomach. This causes the contents of the stomach to reflux into the lower portion of the esophagus, which irritates the cells that line the esophagus. Irritated cells create the burning sensation associated with heartburn.

BEWARE OF CANDY BARS

John Yudkin was studying overweight people and the effect of diets. He noticed that as he cut sugar out of their diets, people with heartburn had less pain. He found this fascinating. So he took seven healthy men and studied their stomach juices. He got a baseline of how much acid these seven men made. Then he put them on a high-sugar diet that was also low in whole grains. Within two weeks, the men's stomachs had started to make 20 percent more acid and pepsin. Yudkin reported his findings in the *British Medical Journal.* He said that too much sugar (sucrose, fructose, and refined cane sugar and syrup), combined with a diet comprised of too little starch (whole grain), promotes unusually high acid production and heartburn.

If you consume just one cola and candy bar a day, you are quadrupling the normal level of blood sugar that your body is evolutionarily set up to manage. Your blood-sugar mechanisms go haywire. This increases your risk of heartburn.

A RASH STOCKBROKER WITH A BURNING HEART

Joe was a stockbroker with a big firm. He suffered with severe heartburn and had to chomp down antacids all day long to relieve the pain. His doctor ran tests and said Joe didn't have an ulcer or any disease or bug. But at night, Joe's burning was so bad that it was scary.

Joe's friend recommended he see me. I interviewed Joe in detail and had him fill out a diet diary and life-stress questionnaire. I told him that his diet and lifestyle had taxed his digestive system. Joe was instructed to do a home-cleansing and rebuilding digestive program, and to take digestive enzymes (stomach acid and pancreatic enzymes) with each meal. Joe also learned how to rub certain reflex points on his feet throughout the day (in between sessions with clients) to strengthen his digestion and elimination. He was given relaxation and meditation tapes to listen to before going to bed to help reduce his stress.

In two months Joe not only had no heartburn, he also had more energy than he'd had for years and a few symptoms he had thought were just part of aging also went away. After that, Joe often couldn't restrain himself from recommending that his clients consider intestinal well-being, not just financial planning.

Health Problems That May Cause Heartburn

If you have *persistent* heartburn, you need to be evaluated by a doctor to rule out some of the possible problems: duodenal and stomach ulcers, heart disease, gallbladder problems, food allergies and/or milk intolerance, and irritable bowel syndrome. If you have heartburn with weight loss, vomiting, loss of appetite, change in eating habits, dark stools, or severe nausea, see a doctor immediately.

Try one or two of the following remedies for *acute* heartburn:

- Drink a glass of water with 2 tablespoons of liquid aloe vera.
- Chew papaya enzymes every 15 minutes for one to two hours.
- Take 1 or 2 deglycyrrhizinated licorice (380 mg) tablets, chewed and swallowed on an empty stomach 20 minutes before meals. (Effectiveness of this substance has not been verified by studies, but clinical reports from doctors such as Gaby and Wright suggest good results.)
- Try slippery elm bark, ginger, or meadowsweet tea.
- Take 2 to 3 capsules several times a day of an antiheartburn formula commercially available at health-food stores. (See appendix B.) If you choose to use a commercial antacid, do it for the short term, not the long term.
- One study suggests that chewing gum causes more saliva, which acts as a natural antacid. But try it for yourself, as some studies say the opposite.
- Try enterically coated peppermint and/or caraway oil—ask your doctor.

Dietary Program for Chronic Heartburn

Try several of the following to see if they reduce heartburn symptoms:

- Rule out infection with *H. pylori* (see chapter 12).
- Evaluate your eating habits and make appropriate changes.
- Identify food allergies.
- Do not drink ice-cold liquids or more than half a glass of liquid with meals.
- Eat more fresh vegetables, whole grains, beans, organic lean turkey, chicken, and fish.
- Eliminate refined sugar (including fructose and corn syrup), refined carbohydrates, colas, caffeine, and alcoholic drinks.
- Avoid chocolate, citrus, tomatoes, onions, peppers, and foods containing peppermint and caffeine.
- Add cultured products or supplements to your diet.
- Lose weight if necessary.
- Doctors used to recommend milk for heartburn, but now we know milk makes the situation worse.

Avoid the Chronic Use of Antacids

In the long run, antacids can make the problem worse, even though they alleviate the symptoms temporarily. They neutralize stomach acid. This interferes with protein absorption and may alter pressure and valve action, creating reflux. This interferes with digestion and can create a stomach environment that encourages the growth of harmful organisms.

Antacid abuse may also cause bone loss. Fourteen cases of bone loss have been reported in the medical literature in women who "abused" antacids for several years.

Antacids are often given to children for reflux and colic, but this can cause rickets and other bone problems.

Supplements for Chronic Heartburn and Gastroesophageal Reflux

Heartburn from drugs? DGL is helpful for patients who must take aspirin, nonsteroidal anti-inflammatory drugs, corticosteroids, and osteoporosis meds. DGL helps reduce heartburn and local irritation that these drugs may cause.

Deglycyrrhizinated licorice (DGL). Chew one or two 380-mg tablets on an empty stomach several times a day. DGL is an herbal preparation of licorice minus the glycyrrhizin (a factor that acts like a hormone). DGL is a safe way to take licorice to help protect the cells that line the stomach and duodenum and to encourage healthy mucus protection.

Friendly bacteria, like *L. acidophilus,* are helpful taken as several capsules two to four times a day.

Aloe vera liquid, several tablespoons to 1/2 cup twice a day. Drink *straight* or add to diluted fruit juice.

Dr. Wright's protocol: If none of the above works, try choline (1 g three times a day), pantothenic acid (500 mg three times a day), manganese citrate (25 mg a day), and vitamin B_1 (250 mg twice a day).

Some people with gastroesophageal reflux actually are low in stomach acid and will need some maintenance hydrochloric acid once the symptoms have gone away, but this should be supervised by a doctor (see chapter 19).

Gallbladder Problems Can Cause Heartburn

It was in 1893 that a doctor first observed that people with gallstones often had too little hydrochloric acid. Since then, numerous research scientists have repeated these studies and come to the same conclusion.

In the article "Gallstones, Gastric Secretion and Flatulent Dyspepsias," in *The Lancet,* the authors, English surgeons, discuss how heartburn and gas often go along with too little stomach acid (hydrochloric acid). They frequently saw gallbladder patients who had heartburn and gas, but proved to also have inadequate levels of stomach acid.

Some of you with a history of gallbladder illness may experience improved health and less heartburn by taking digestive supplements. How many of you were ever told this?

Treatment for Hiatal Hernia

A hiatal hernia occurs when a portion of your stomach actually slides up abnormally above the diaphragm. Forty percent of people who have been X-rayed have been found to have hiatal hernia. Some of these people experience heartburn and digestive discomfort and others don't have symptoms.

What to Do:
- Lose weight.
- Improve posture.
- Sleep with the head of your bed several inches higher than your feet.
- Avoid overeating.
- Do not eat several hours before going to bed.
- Don't eat after exercising.
- Do not drink more than one-half glass of fluids with your meals for two weeks. Then keep it down to one beverage per meal.
- Avoid bending over after eating, as much as possible. In other words, do not eat and then go out and weed your garden or stand on your head.
- Avoid ice-cold drinks and foods, or consume sparingly.
- Identify food allergies.

What to Take for Hiatal Hernia:
- **Deglycyrrhizinated licorice (DGL)**, 1 or 2 tablets, chewed and swallowed on empty stomach twice day, 20 minutes before meals. Take for several months.
- **Vitamin B$_1$,** 200 mg once a day with a backup B complex.
- **Cultured dairy products** (see chapter 3).
- **Digestive enzymes,** if appropriate (see chapter 19).

Hands-on Help

See a chiropractor, osteopath, or massage person who knows how to perform "soft tissue" manipulation for this problem. I have seen hands-on methods (downward manual pressure and traction applied by practitioners who know what they are doing) to be helpful in controlling, if not eliminating, this condition, when accompanied by proper exercise and dietary suggestions.

Juices and Foods for Heartburn, Reflux, and Hiatal Hernia

Freely consume the items below for two weeks. These foods and teas are soothing and healing to the upper intestinal tract.

Cooling juice. Juice cucumbers and celery and dilute with water; a little yogurt or kefir is optional.

Cooling teas. Chamomile tea with 1 teaspoon of chlorophyll added, or tea from slippery elm bark steeped with ginger and fennel.

Cooling shakes. Thoroughly blend half a banana, diluted apple juice, and several almonds with water.

Cooling soups. Zucchini soup: steam zucchini and blend with the water the vegetables were steamed in. Add a little butter and sea salt.

Cucumber soup. Blend peeled cucumbers with yogurt and dill.

Cooling snacks. Yogurt mixed with organic applesauce. Flavored kefir blended with ground seeds.

Cooling meals. Millet and steamed vegetables. Brown rice and sautéed zucchini. Brown or Chinese black rice cooked with mung beans and buckwheat groats. Salads that have fresh sprouts, especially sunflower, and grated root vegetables (beets, Jerusalem artichoke, celery root, jicama).

Mind-Body Techniques

Reflex Points for Heartburn Relief

Sit in a relaxed position. With your thumb, push up the ball of your foot under your big toe. Find the sorest spot on the ball of your foot and hold it tightly with your thumb. Feel for painful or gritty areas. Run your knuckles down the sides of your lower legs, working out sore spots. Even though these are unconventional points for this problem, clinically I have found them to be helpful. (See foot charts at the end of chapter 20.)

Affirmation for Heartburn

Inhale and visualize drawing this breath into the stomach.
Exhale and visualize the breath relaxing the stomach.
With each *inhale* say, *"I relax my stomach."*

With each *exhale* say, "*My stomach is cooling.*"
Repeat as many times as you want.

Exercises for Heartburn

1. *Cooling Pose and Affirmation*—to be done when you are actively experiencing heartburn:

Lie on your back with a thin pillow under your shoulder blades. This opens up your chest. Place your hands over the area where you feel burning. Inhale and exhale three times to get relaxed.

Now, with your eyes closed, visualize breathing cool blue light in through your nostrils into your upper chest. On the exhale, visualize the cooling light *coating* your stomach.

On the *inhale* say, "*Draw in.*"
On the *exhale* say, "*Cooling.*"
On the *inhale* say, "*Draw in.*"
On the *exhale* say, "*Healing.*" Relax.
Repeat as often as comfortable. Then relax.

2. *Modified Cobra Pose for Upper Intestines and Valve*—to be done to prevent heartburn when you are not having it:

Lie on your stomach with your hands flat on the floor near your shoulders. Inhale and press your hands against the floor to gently lift your head and upper body off the floor as far as possible but without straining as you look upward. Maintaining this position, exhale, and feel as though you can stretch your torso away from your waist. The sensation is that you are tractioning your upper body away from the lower portion of your body.

Imagine your intestinal tract is getting a healthy stretch deep inside. Stay in this position for several deep breaths, then slowly come down. Repeat three times and do this daily for two weeks. Hold your abdomen and buttocks firm while doing this to avoid straining your back.

Meditation for Heartburn

Sit or lie quietly in a relaxed position. Become aware of your mouth. Notice how your mouth feels. Extend your awareness to your esophagus and into your stomach. Notice how they feel. Now extend your awareness into your stomach. How does your stomach and the lining of your stomach feel?

In your mind's eye, visualize drawing in healing, cooling blue light with your breath. Draw this light, with your inhale, into your nose. Let this cooling blue light travel down into your stomach. Let it cool and relax the walls of your stomach. On the exhale, see the blue light leave your stomach and fill the rest of your body. Let the exhale carry this healing light throughout your body. Visualize the blue light coming out of all your pores, so you are surrounded by blue light. Inhale the blue light and, on the exhale be surrounded by blue light. Once you have this visualization firmly in your mind's eye (blue inside and out), sit quietly in the midst of this cooling sensation for five to ten minutes. Take nine deep breaths before you get up. Notice how different your mouth, esophagus, and stomach feel.

Mindful Living

Since the importance of communication is now appreciated, let's extend this to our bodies. If you have heartburn, this may be a "signal" that some detail of your life needs to be heard. Reread the list of common causes of heartburn and see what may apply to you.

7 *Causes and Treatments of Constipation*

Constipation is anything but romantic. We never imagine screen idols who are hugging sexy costars to be privately constipated. But constipation happens to the best of us and, if you're constipated, it's hard to be romantic, energetic, or fully enjoy your life.

As you recall, elimination is an essential point on the digestive triangle. Constipation can mean a decreased frequency of bowel movements or a normal number of inadequately small bowel movements. Small, dry, and hard stools, even if eliminated once or twice a day, are not optimal elimination.

Inadequate elimination puts a burden on the intestinal tract, the internal bacterial balance (intestinal ecology), and the cells of the intestinal lining. Also, drier than normal stools often require straining and squeezing, which puts a further burden on the lower tissues of the intestinal tract. Constipation, if continued over a period of time, can put a strain on the liver, as well as on the rest of the body.

JOAN'S HEADACHES LINKED TO HER CONSTIPATION

Joan was a hardworking single mom who suffered from chronic headaches for over five years. Physical therapy, chiropractic, and acupuncture had all failed to relieve her pain. Joan was losing sleep, becoming depressed, and having a harder time being patient with her little daughter. A close friend who was a pharmacist told her of one client who got rid of his headaches by treating his constipation.

Joan was amazed. She frequently had trouble moving her bowels, but she hadn't linked this to her headaches. Then and there, Joan decided to tackle her constipation. She drank more water and improved her eating habits. She started to eat more green vegetables and fruit and added whole grains to her evening meal. Her pharmacist friend recommended magnesium. Joan also started walking briskly through a mall, with her daughter in a stroller, three or four times a week.

In one month Joan was eliminating one or two times a day, whereas previously she used to go only once a week. Two weeks later her headaches stopped. Joan would be the first to admit that "everything's connected."

An Important Connection

The idea that constipation and poor elimination are the cause of many diseases, including premature aging, was first introduced in the early 1900s by the Nobel Prize–winning Russian biologist Elie Metchnikoff. In the last several decades, Drs. Bernard Jensen, Paavo Airola, Jonathan Wright, Alan Gaby, Leo Galland, Martin Lee, and Jeff Bland's teachings to thousands of health-care professionals, based on the scientific literature and the treating of thousands of medical patients, has furthered the respect for this link.

Even though you may still run into doctors who don't accept this connection between intestinal and total health, both scientific studies and clinical experiences are demonstrating the vital importance of a healthy bowel to overall health. New holistic laboratory procedures examine stool to evaluate digestion. Old terms like "colon hygiene" may be laughed at, but the concept of digestive health isn't.

What Is Normal or Not

A healthy person should have at least one bowel movement a day. Medical textbooks state that individual variation goes from several times a day to several times a week. However, having worked with people for many years on improving their health, I would define constipation as not having one to several daily bowel movements, or having too long an intestinal-transit time. Transit time is how long food takes to go from your mouth through your intestines. One bowel movement a day with an excessively long intestinal-transit time is still constipation. Chapter 1 guides you through easy self-assessment of your intestinal-transit time.

I consistently observed that individuals who didn't eliminate daily had more health problems, especially fatigue, gas, bloating, abdominal discomfort, predisposition to skin conditions, allergies, anxiety, depression, headaches, female disorders, insomnia, and less mental energy. They also often healed more slowly. It's hard to feel your best if waste products are not being cleared efficiently out of your system.

Severe constipation is eliminating every several days or once or twice a week.

What's Normal for You?

Referring to "usual" bowel habits means how your bowels move *most of the time.* If you have problems every once in a while, for example, after a dietary indiscretion, this is not a concern. However, if during most of the month you have hard stools, can't easily eliminate, pass little pellet-sized stools, have abdominal pain or alternating bouts of hard stools with diarrhea, then something is wrong.

Remember, your stools—their frequency, appearance, smell, color, and the presence or absence of undigested food—are an excellent indication of how your gastrointestinal tract is doing.

Easy Evaluation of Your Elimination

Your stools should:

- Be full and round, sometimes float, and be somewhat long in length.
- Be medium to dark brown.
- Be easily passed and "feel" complete. Straining, squeezing, or having to sit for a long time for anything to happen are signs the digestive tract is not working optimally.
- Not smell bad.
- Not be accompanied by blood caused by irritation or tearing of rectal tissues.
- Not be greasy, or be oily with lots of bubbles.
- Not be in hard little pieces, or thin little tubes as though they were squeezed out of a toothpaste tube (these are signs of intestinal spasms—cramping of the muscular lining of the intestines).

You should feel comfortable, empty, and a little energetic or relieved after a good bowel movement.

Constipation Is a Red Flag

Persistent constipation is a signal that you need to evaluate your life habits and *fix* something. Your diet may have too many refined foods and not enough fiber; you may not be exercising enough; you may be eating and living at a hectic pace; you may not be drinking enough water; you may be stressed-out; you may be deficient in certain nutrients; your thyroid may be underactive; or you may be overeating nutrient-poor foods or foods to which you are allergic.

Most of the effects of constipation occur because waste materials are left inside your intestinal tract for much longer than is optimal. When this goes on for extended periods of time, the risk of various problems is enhanced. Toxic "particles" can be created that can damage digestive enzymes in your intestinal

A slow transit time increases reabsorption of bile, which increases cholesterol levels. One way to lower cholesterol is to improve your intestinal transit time.

wall and thus cause maldigestion and nutrient deficiencies. The walls of your colon can weaken, which can create hernias in the wall, called *diverticulosis*.

Excessive transit time can contribute to colitis, irritable bowel syndrome, and lower intestinal pain. When waste becomes drier, harder, and more difficult to eliminate, stress is put on your rectum, which can cause rectal disease and hemorrhoids. Excessive transit time also promotes the growth of unfriendly bacteria. These unfriendly bacteria can act on the waste to create cancer-causing and health-debilitating substances that can get reabsorbed into your body.

One hormone potentially affected by constipation is estrogen. Studies suggest constipation may indirectly cause estrogen to be reabsorbed. The increased exposure to this hormone may elevate the risk of estrogen-dependent problems, ranging from painful breasts and PMS to more severe problems, such as endometriosis, infertility, and breast cancer. Future research will probably show that many hormones are affected.

In *The Lancet* (November 28, 1991), one study compared the rate of bowel movements with the risk of breast disease. Normal and abnormal cells in the breast fluid collected from 1,481 women were studied. Women with daily bowel movements had a 5.1 percent rate of abnormal (dysplastic) cells. Women with two or less bowel movements a week had 23.2 percent abnormal cells.

The authors concluded that daily bowel movements probably help maintain normal estrogen levels in women. Elevated levels of estrogen throughout a woman's life increase her risk of infertility, breast cancer, and other cancers. Thus, constipation is a female adversary, whereas regular bowel movements are a woman's ally.

Excessive transit time puts a stress on other digestive organs (gallbladder, pancreas, and liver). This can cause problems such as fatigue and headaches. Excessive transit time and prolonged exposure to waste products can create changes in gas pressure that reflux food backward. This can damage your esophagus. Gases can rise upward, irritating throat, gums, tongue, and teeth, and cause bad breath. These gases can make you feel ill physically and mentally.

Prolonged and severe constipation can create vulnerabilities to liver problems, varicose veins, arthritis, and lower back pain, as well as put a burden on your immune system.

Five Lifestyle Treatments for Constipation

1. *Exercise.* Lack of sufficient physical exercise is the most commonly overlooked cause of constipation. You need to move in order to help your intestinal tract keep moving. Humans used to walk everywhere. Now we drive everywhere. In this way, constipation is one side effect of the automobile.

   Evolutionarily speaking, our bodies are set up to be moving much of the day. To make up for the fact we don't move much anymore, we *have to* fit in some regular form of exercise.

Try 1 tablespoon flaxseed oil on hot cereal or ground flaxseeds in yogurt, in salad, or just in a spoon. Add extra-virgin olive oil in salad dressing or on food, or use as "Italian butter" for dunking your bread.

When you add regular physical exercise into your life, you will tone up the muscles in your arms, legs, lungs, and heart. This exercises your intestinal muscular wall and promotes the manufacture of Glutamine that helps feed intestinal-lining cells. Exercise also decreases anxiety, which is another contributor to constipation. (Anxiety can cause harder *or* looser stools, depending on the individual.)

2. *Eat more fiber foods.* We in the West do not like to change our diets. We'd rather take quick, easy fixes, such as pills and powders. We have translated this newly recognized need for fiber into powders, bran supplements, and refined foods with bran added. These are helpful but they are not real whole foods. *There is no substitute for "real" foods* like whole grains, dark-green vegetables, raw nuts, sprouts, and seeds—all of which contain excellent fiber, nutrients, and oils, and act as natural lubricants.

3. *Liquids.* Dehydration is an overlooked cause of constipation. Drink plenty of liquids—five to eight glasses per day of filtered water, herbal tea, and *diluted* fruit juices (fruit juices straight from the bottle, even "sugar-free" fruit juices, are high in sugars and play havoc with the delicate lining of your intestinal tract). Many of us overconsume excessively sugared drinks and salty foods, which dehydrate us.

4. *Quality lubricants.* Oils have a lubricating effect on the mucous walls of the colon. Avoid hydrogenated and processed oils, which do not do the job as well as natural olive and seed oils do.

5. *Eat more fruit and cultured food products.* Add two to three fresh fruits a day into your diet, such as apples, pears, pineapple, or papaya. Fruits contain water, fiber, and natural vitamins and minerals that assist intestinal transit time. Soak dried fruits, like figs (try both black mission and calymira) or prunes, and mix with yogurt (labeled as containing live cultures) and have some at night as a healthy snack. This fruit mixture is also tasty over hot cereal in the morning. Get organic dried fruits whenever possible, because drying concentrates pesticides and chemicals in the food.

Add cultured products several times a week, if not daily. Cultured products like yogurt and kefir contain friendly microorganisms that optimize intestinal transit time. If you are an allergic or reactive person, don't have cow's-milk products on a daily basis. Try eating them one to three times a week, depending on the degree of your sensitivity, and try other cultured sources like Dilly Beans (pickled string beans) or soy yogurt.

Meat: A Fiberless Food

Meat is a very constipating food because it has no fiber, it takes a long time to move through the colon, and it promotes the growth of putrefying bacteria. This does not mean that you should not eat meat. Some people require meat to feel fit. But you should not *overeat* meat. Your diet should be *balanced* among vegetables, fruits, beans, seeds, whole grains, and meats.

Common food allergies, such as cheese, for example, can also be constipating in sensitive individuals.

Natural Answers for *Acute* Constipation

Milk is the most common allergic food causing constipation, especially in children.

Before bed, try one to two of the items listed below. People who eat plenty of fiber and still have constipation should also try the following:

For Acute Constipation

- *Flaxseed oil.* 1 tablespoon by itself or mixed with a little cultured cottage cheese, yogurt, and/or honey.
- *Magnesium.* 250 mg once or twice a day.
- *Vitamin C.* 1 gram, twice a day.
- *Cascara sagrada.* 2 to 4 capsules before bed. This herb stimulates peristalsis of the intestinal tract (muscular action). Do not take this herb for more than ten days.

Specific Foods for Constipation

Fruit Smoothies   Blend a cut-up apple, diluted apple juice, and a handful of raw almonds with the skins left on. Optional: Add one teaspoon of ground-up flaxseed.

Blend an apple and diluted fruit juice with The Ultimate Meal (can be purchased at health-food stores) or some other excellent protein/high-fiber source.

Cultured Cottage Cheese Delights   Soak dried black mission figs and dried cherries overnight in hot water. Add to cultured cottage cheese, shredded carrots, and diced apples. Serve over lettuce.

Add diced apples and 1 tablespoon of flaxseed oil to cultured cottage cheese. Optional: Sprinkle tamarind pumpkin seeds on top.

Fruit Cereal   Soak black mission figs overnight. Add to either cold or hot cereal.

Fresh Vegetables   Eat more greens and darker greens. If you don't like them or if they aren't available, make a green drink (see page 53). If you don't want to do this, at least take commercially available capsules or powders made from greens, algae, or other chlorophyll sources.

Tasty Greens   Put a little water and 1 teaspoon of olive oil in a pan. Add a large amount of spinach, cover, and heat. This cooks the spinach somewhere between steaming and sautéing. Serve with a little lemon juice or balsamic vinegar and a bit more olive oil or butter (raw, unsalted) to taste. You can use the same method for chard, collard greens, beet greens, and kale.

Tasty Broccoli   Cut up broccoli. Put in a saucepan with a little water and olive oil. Heat. Add several tablespoons (to taste) of either hoisin sauce or plum sauce (available in the Oriental food section of your supermarket). Optional: Dice garlic and sprinkle over top for the last several minutes of cooking. Serve over rice with strips of any of the following: chicken, lamb, tofu, tempeh, or seitan.

Other Food Ideas for Constipation

Buy whole flaxseeds, keep refrigerated, grind in coffee grinder, and sprinkle on cereals and salads. Tastes nutty.

Use a blend of 2/3 olive oil and 1/3 flaxseed oil to make salad dressings. Add balsamic vinegar, soy sauce. Optional: Blend in a little mustard, garlic and/or horseradish.

Use more garlic in cooking. Garlic contains allicin, a unique substance that stimulates the muscular action of the walls of the intestinal tract.

Soak black mission figs overnight. Blend with vanilla yogurt and water. Or eat figs whole over yogurt.

Eat whole berries on top of yogurt, or mix together in a blender.

Juices for Constipation

Morning Move   Juice fresh oranges, lemons, grapefruit (and pineapple if you have it). Drink this or pour on top of whole-grain cereal instead of milk.

Afternoon Move   Juice garlic, tomato, onion, and carrot. Optional, add beet greens, spinach, parsley, or celery.

Green Drink   See page 53.

Helpful Supplements for Chronic Constipation

- *A high-quality multiple vitamin/mineral* and a B complex once a day enhances bowel regularity for some folks. If this helps, stay on this as maintenance. If a multivitamin/mineral does not help, consider implementing *one of the following suggestions for two weeks and if that doesn't work, try the next one, or any that seems appropriate for you.*
- Try *fiber cocktails.* (see chapter 2, page 25).
- *Note:* A very few people are allergic or hypersensitive to psyllium. These sensitive folks may get more constipated or develop some allergic manifestation, such as canker sores or allergic shiners (dark rings under the eyes).
- *Magnesium,* 250 to 800 mg a day, in divided dosages. If you take more than you need, you may get loose stools. If this happens, just cut back the dosage until your stools firm up.

Note: Magnesium is hydrophilic. This means that it draws water into the bowel. This makes magnesium a natural stool softener. Inadequate levels of magnesium are a common cause of constipation. Magnesium is rinsed out of the body during stress and it is easily deficient in a diet with inadequate green vegetables. This is because magnesium is at the center of the chlorophyll molecule. Chlorophyll capsules are an excellent natural source of magnesium.

Four signs that suggest inadequate magnesium tissue levels are: constipation, muscle cramps and/or twitches, body odor, and an increased startle reflex to noises.

- *Flaxseed oil,* 1 tablespoon twice a day. (If you have trouble, such as nausea, burping, or bloating, take the oil with digestive enzymes containing bile salts for several weeks.)
- *Digestive enzymes.* Insufficient levels of digestive enzymes—hydrochloric acid, pancreatic enzymes, and bile salts—can cause constipation. See chapter 19 to help you assess whether digestive enzyme insufficiency applies to you.

  Nutritional alternatives to digestive enzymes include sipping water mixed with 1 teaspoon apple-cider vinegar and 1 teaspoon honey—or with the juice of a fresh lemon—throughout a meal. If you think you need some bile stimulation, natural alternatives are supplements with Black Russian radish powder, beet powder, urva ursi, yellow dock, or milk thistle.
- *Folic acid,* 400 mg daily. Folic acid deficiency has been linked to constipation, and it is very difficult to get adequate amounts from our diet.
- *Aloe vera juice,* 1/3 cup mixed with water or juice before bed and on rising.
- *Thiamine (B₁),* 100 to 300 mg once a day.

More options:

- *L. acidophilus,* 2 to 3 capsules twice daily, or eat cultured foods such as yogurt.

  Note: Laxative abuse (associated with eating disorders) may ultimately cause constipation. So may other medications or iron supplements (natural heme forms of iron, such as iron peptonate, do not have as irritating and constipating an effect as do the other forms of iron). If you have been abusing laxatives, take some probiotics (3 to 4 capsules three to four times a day for at least two months) and consider a complete stool workup by a professional. New stool tests can tell how well you're digesting foods and your ratio of friendly to unfriendly bacteria.
- *Inositol* is part of the vitamin B complex. It helps stimulate the muscular wall of the intestinal tract. Inadequate inositol in the body can be associated with constipation. Too much caffeine rinses the body of inositol. Inositol is

found in unrefined whole grains, citrus fruits, and brewer's yeast. Take 100 to 300 mg a day.

- *Pantothenic acid,* 500 mg to 3 grams before bed. Insufficient pantothenic acid (B₅) can contribute to constipation. Pantothenic acid is essential for optimal intestinal functioning. It helps some postoperative patients who experience slow transit time, gas pains, and distention.

Healing Herbs for Constipation

Acute herbs get you moving when you are constipated, but are not to be taken for extended periods of time. *Maintenance herbs* are to be taken for one month to tone the intestinal tract.

Acute Herbs   Make a strong tea or purchase commercial formulas that contain any of the following: cascara sagrada, senna leaf or pod, sarsaparilla, urva ursi, goldenseal, mountain flax, buckthorn bark, dandelion, slippery elm, or alder.

Drink tea three times a day or take 2 capsules two or three times a day before meals as needed.

Maintenance Herbs   Make a strong brew of peppermint with a small amount of licorice. Steep for ten minutes. Drink 1 cup before going to bed, with 1 teaspoon of liquid chlorophyll. Take for one month.

If Your Stools Smell Bad

If you have malodorous stools, rule out bacterial or parasitic infections (see chapter 15), then try one or two of the following:

- *L. acidophilus* and other helpful microorganisms for one month upon rising and before going to bed. Take 2 or 3 capsules or 1 teaspoon in water.
- *Magnesium* and/or a green drink (see page 53).
- *Digestive enzymes* if you need them (see chapter 19).
- *Herbs:* Mix 1/3 teaspoon each of powdered ginger, fennel, and turmeric with unprocessed honey and eat with a spoon, followed by warm water or tea. This also helps halitosis.

Avoiding Constipation While Traveling or in New Situations

Try one or two of the following hints.

- Take multidigestive enzymes with each meal. If traveling, start taking them several days before you leave. *Note:* Don't take if you have any kind of ulcers.
- Take two capsules of *L. acidophilus* and *bifidus* before bedtime, or consume yogurt daily.

- Before bed, take 100 mgs of inositol, 250 mg magnesium, and 1 gram of vitamin C.
- Try commercial herbal formulas for constipation before bed (see appendix B).

For Persistent Constipation

Identify and eliminate food allergies (see chapter 18).

If your constipation is due to *parasites*, nothing may work, or you may experience only slight improvement until you eradicate the parasites. Customary stool labs may not detect parasites adequately (see chapter 15).

Low thyroid (hypothyroid) may be associated with chronic constipation. You may need to get checked for hypothyroidism or subclinical hypothyroidism, with blood work and body temperature, by a doctor who is familiar with Dr. Broda Barnes's work. Dr. Barnes suggested that the average blood test doesn't pick up subclinical hypothyroidism, and discovered that a below-normal body temperature is a more sensitive indicator of low thyroid, along with other clinical symptoms.

Important: If You've Had Constipation for a Long Time

If you have had a history of being constipated for three months or longer, you should add some nutritional liver support for two months. The liver gets overworked from having to detoxify the same substances multiple times.

Take milk thistle in capsules (2 or 3) or in high-quality liquid tinctures (1/3 dropper), twice a day for two months. If you have had constipation for years, add the same amount of yellow dock for several weeks to a month. Also, consider a bowel detoxification and rebuilding program (see chapter 20).

Sometimes lifelong constipation is associated with a history of early sexual abuse, which creates a disconnection from one's body; in such cases, therapy should be part of the healing process.

Mind-Body Techniques

Three Exercises for Intestinal Toning for Constipation

1. *Stomach flapping.* Do this 25 times on rising and before going to bed. (See chapter 2, page 30.)
2. *Baby pose.* Sit on your heels on the floor, lean forward until your forehead touches the ground, and relax like this for several minutes. Put your arms by

your side. Gently inhale and exhale. This simple position gently stimulates and relaxes your intestinal tract.

3. *Abdominal windmill.* Lie on your back. Bring your knees up to your chest. Place both knees to your right, touching the floor on your right side. Then, keeping your knees together, revolve to the left, touching the floor on your left side. If you need to, hold your knees together with your hands, and if you need to help move your knees with your hands, do so. Repeat 10 to 20 times. Relax. Do two sets only after you have done one set a day for one week.

Reflex Points for Constipation

With knuckles, rub up and down on the center of the foot along the area of the digestive tract. (See the end of chapter 20 for foot reflexology charts.) With your fingers, try to find sore spots. Work out the sore spots or any gritty nodules that you feel. Work the ball of the right foot first, then the left. Finish by stimulating or pressing up the outside of the right foot and across the instep, then across the instep of the left foot to the outside and then down to the heel. Repeat this move three times using both feet.

Be near a bathroom. Sometimes the effects are immediate.

Intestinal Fist Massage

Your intestinal tract runs up your right side, across the top (under your rib cage), and down your left side. Lie on your back. Bend your knees with your feet on the floor by your buttocks. Focus on your abdomen. Relax this area. Inhale, letting your breath fill up your abdomen, and stretch it toward the ceiling. Hold this breath and stretch your abdomen further. Then, with your exhale, let your abdomen sink gently into your body. Do three of these breaths.

Holding your hands in very gentle partial fists, rub your abdominal area in tiny circles. Rub in this pattern: up your right side, across the top (under your ribs), and down your left side. Repeat three to ten times. Finish with three more full breaths. See page 31 for the pattern of massage on abdomen. This exercise, however, uses fists, that one uses the fingers.

8 Easy Treatments for Diarrhea

Diarrhea is frequent passage, usually involuntarily, of unformed or watery stools. Feces are normally made up of about three-fourths water and one-forth solid matter. With diarrhea, the water content is higher. What causes diarrhea is irritation and/or increased motility (muscular activity) inside your intestinal tract. This can be due to a varying number of possibilities, from nutrient deficiencies to infections from various bugs. Thus, diarrhea is actually a symptom of some kind of intestinal problem.

ZINC DEFICIENCY AND DIARRHEA

Five-year-old Cindy, from a poor family, suffered from repeated episodes of diarrhea, as well as chronic respiratory problems. Her mother used over-the-counter drugs, then took Cindy to a clinic that put her on prescription drugs. But as soon as Cindy stopped taking anything, her problems returned.

One day a nutritionist was giving a free clinic at a local grocery store. The nutritionist noted that Cindy's nails had white spots on them. Also, when asked, Cindy admitted that she was addicted to sweets. These two signs suggested that Cindy may have had a zinc deficiency. The nutritionist recommended Cindy take zinc, in tablet form, once a day. At first Cindy got an upset stomach. So the nutritionist reduced the dose. Within several days, Cindy felt better. Within several weeks, her diarrhea ended. Over several months, Cindy's overall health improved.

There are two types of diarrhea: *acute,* a one-time episode caused by a temporary problem, and *chronic,* a persistent condition of usually five or more watery stools a day, signaling an ongoing problem. Your job is to sleuth out the irritating cause.

Diarrhea often comes with other symptoms: abdominal bloating, abdominal pain, intestinal rumbling and noises (*borborygmi*—yes, I know, try to say *that* three times), loss of appetite, increased thirst, and a sore rectum from frequent elimination.

If blood and mucus are present, something more serious may be going on. You must be evaluated by a doctor if you have blood or mucus in your stool, if another family member also had diarrhea when you did, if the diarrhea persists and is nonresponsive to home treatments, if you have fever over 101°F, or if you have *severe* pain in your abdomen or rectum.

Causes of Acute (Short Attack) Diarrhea

Antibiotic therapy. Antibiotics can kill off the friendly bacteria in your gastrointestinal tract, which allows the unfriendly bacteria to become too numerous, which in turn can irritate your insides and create toxicity. Other medications may also cause diarrhea.

Sugar intolerances. The most common sugars that cause diarrhea-type problems are: milk sugar, hexitol, sorbitol, and mannitol sugars, which are used as sugar substitutes in dietetic foods, candies, and gums. Sugar intolerances to these are called "dietetic food" or "chewing-gum" diarrhea. Sorbitol occurs naturally in many foods that are known for their laxative properties. Apple juice and pear nectars also cause trouble in some sensitive children and adults. When you stop eating these foods the symptoms may go away immediately or take a whole night to calm down.

Vitamin C or magnesium. High levels can cause diarrhea.

Bouts of emotional *stress* and anxiety.

Poorly absorbed *salts,* such as magnesium sulfates and sodium phosphates, cause irritation to your intestinal tract, which can cause diarrhea.

Parasitic infections. Often, the first sign of infection by a parasite is diarrhea, which may be accompanied by pain and fever. Sometimes chronic diarrhea may suggest undetected parasite infections. Some parasite infections elude normal stool tests. If you have diarrhea with fever and/or a rash, you should see a doctor.

Laxatives may cause diarrhea, and abuse of laxatives may cause a chronic problem with diarrhea, poor absorption, and damage to the lining of the intestinal tract, which may adversely affect overall health.

Unfriendly bacteria. Consuming food or water under poor sanitary conditions can lead to contamination, most commonly by toxigenic *E. coli.* The resulting diarrhea is often called "Montezuma's Revenge" or "turista."

Radiation or chemotherapies can kill off the friendly bacteria in the intestinal tract.

Viral infections. The Rotavirus and Norwalk virus are the most common causes of acute diarrhea in children under two years old.

Food Poisoning. Diarrhea from food poisoning usually occurs within half an hour to a day after eating contaminated food. Symptoms are diarrhea, nausea, abdominal pain, and vomiting, which usually last for one-half to a whole day. Suspect this if several people who consumed the same food are affected. Severe cases need a doctor.

What to Do for *Acute* Diarrhea

- *Stop eating your regular food.* You need to rest your intestinal tract. This is essential. What you eat will not get properly digested, and it will add to your already toxic load.
- *Don't take commercial medications* that stop the diarrhea, because diarrhea is your body's effort to throw off what is irritating your intestinal tract. Do take gentle herbal remedies.
- *Drink plenty of fluids,* as it is easy to get dehydrated. Be especially watchful of dehydration in children. Drink teas (chamomile, raspberry, slippery elm, or ginger), sip carob powder stirred in hot water, drink green drinks (see page 53), or sip a cup of water with 1 teaspoon of chlorophyll in it.
- *Make diluted rice water.* Boil 1 cup of rice with 4 cups of water for 45 minutes, strain, add salt until it tastes pleasantly salty to you, and drink half a cup from five to seven times throughout the day. This is excellent for soothing your intestinal tract and getting some easily absorbed nutrients.
- *Consume yogurt* with bananas or cooked applesauce and several teaspoons of fiber. This is soothing and is high in pectin, which calms the intestinal tract and supplies nutrients that diarrhea rinses out—magnesium and potassium.

Do items 1 or 2 below, depending on what you have available, then add the rest of the list.

1. Take 4 charcoal tablets every hour for several hours, and then reduce to three times a day for two more days, or until the diarrhea stops. (This makes stools *black* for several days.) Do not take charcoal with food or vitamins. If you don't have charcoal, you can try well-charred pieces of toast.
2. Try 2 or 3 capsules of commercial soothing gastric formulas every hour on an empty stomach until the diarrhea calms down (see appendix B). These are available at health-food stores. Reduce dosage to several times a day, between meals, for one or two more days when the diarrhea has stopped.
3. Take potassium (99 mg) and a multimineral (ideally in liquid form).
4. Take 3 to 4 capsules of probiotics three to four times a day. If you don't have this, eat generous amounts of yogurt that contains live probiotics. If you are allergic to dairy products, try soy yogurt. Continue taking 2 capsules twice a day and consuming cultured products for one to two weeks after having diarrhea.

Other Alternatives

- Try 1/2 teaspoon of the following; roasted carob powder, turmeric powder, and cinnamon twice daily, mixed with water or tea. If you only have one of these, use that. Mix in unprocessed honey, if you like.
- One cup of liquid aloe vera one to two times a day away from food.
- *Saccharomyces boulardii* is a nonpathogenic yeast originally isolated from the surface of lichee nuts. It has been used in Europe to treat diarrhea. This is good to take while traveling to both treat and prevent traveler's diarrhea. You can purchase it at your health-food store.

Food Tips for When Acute Diarrhea Starts to Subside

- Slowly reintroduce small amounts of foods.
- Avoid dairy products and raw fruits, vegetables, and salads for several days.
- Avoid refined sugars and alcoholic beverages. Don't drink soda pop. Add water or carbonated water to a small amount of fruit juice, or unfiltered honey to tea.
- Consume high-fiber foods like cereals, bran muffins, and lots of cultured food.

Possible Causes of Chronic (Ongoing) Diarrhea

Diseases of the colon. Colitis (inflammation of the intestinal wall), irritable bowel syndrome (intestinal disorders with pain but no sign of organic disease), diverticulitis (inflammation of small herniations of the colon), and colon cancer can cause diarrhea. See a doctor to rule these out.

Caffeinated beverages. Coffee, tea, colas, chocolate, and many over-the-counter drugs may contain caffeine, and daily caffeine consumption may be contributing to your problem. Very sensitive folks may be affected by only one cup of coffee a day. Go off caffeinated beverages for a week and see if you improve.

Nutrient deficiencies. Low level of nutrients that normally protect the intestinal lining and gastrointestinal tract may cause diarrhea. Zinc is the most common culprit. Also possibly involved are A and B vitamins and glutamine.

Stomach acid. Your stomach may not make enough hydrochloric acid. One of the common signs of low stomach acid is chronic early morning loose stools or diarrhea, or recurrent flatulence immediately after eating.

Food allergies, the most common being to wheat or milk, can cause diarrhea. Go off both for two weeks, then reintroduce one at a time and see what happens. According to Dr. James Breneman, chronic diarrhea is a frequent sign of food allergy. Dr. Breneman says, "It is so frequent, in fact, that the most effective single method of diarrhea control is food allergy exclusion."

Unfriendly bacteria, candida, or parasitic infections. One study in Italy identified "dead yeast" in people with chronic diarrhea. If regular stool tests don't identify a pathogen, try a stool test that requires several samples over several different days.

Celiac disease. Rule out a genetic inability to digest *gluten*, which is found in wheat, oats, barley, and rye. This problem is called *celiac disease*. In sensitive people, gliadin, a fraction of gluten, can damage the intestinal lining and cause diarrhea as well as blood loss and anemia. Go off all gluten products for one month. Then add these back in large amounts and see what happens. Gas, abdominal cramping, light-colored stools, canker sores, and fatigue suggest difficulty digesting gluten. If going off these foods does not reduce your diarrhea, gluten sensitivity is most likely not your problem. If it is, substitute gluten grains with corn, quinoa, brown rice, spelt, and amaranth. Sometimes millet and buckwheat will not cause problems. You have to explore and see which grains agree with you.

Subclinical celiac disease. New studies suggest more people than previously thought suffer from this. These people may get symptoms on and off—depending on stress, how often gluten foods are consumed, and other digestive and lifestyle factors. If someone in your family has celiac disease, you have a higher risk of this.

New diet. Have you been overzealous in your attempts to cleanse your GI tract or to add fiber? Look at how you have changed your life in the past several weeks. See if you can figure out something you have been doing that is contributing to your problem.

Local irritation caused by excessive alcohol, sugar, salt, food additives, aspirin, NSAIDs (nonsteroidal anti-inflammatory medication), or nicotine exposure. Some individuals are more sensitive than others.

Laxative abuse.

Sensitive reactions to *food additives and colorings*. Strictly avoid these in your diet and see if your diarrhea goes away.

Pellagra, a niacin deficiency, causes the 3 D's—diarrhea, dermatitis, and dementia. Niacin deficiency can contribute to chronic diarrhea. Other vitamin B deficiencies can aggravate or cause diarrhea tendencies, especially folic acid and vitamin B_1 deficiencies.

Tips for *Chronic* Diarrhea

Do everything noted under acute diarrhea, but don't stop eating. Also follow the guidelines below.

Avoid caffeinated beverages and raw foods. Avoid highly allergic foods like cow's-milk product products, beef, and gluten. Don't eat processed fats or refined sugar.

Consume plenty of steamed vegetables and cultured products several times a day. Sip teas and carob drinks throughout the day.

Identify and eliminate food allergies (see chapter 18). Check for fungal or parasitic infections (see chapter 15). Check to see if you require digestive enzymes (see chapter 19). Learn stress-coping skills, if appropriate.

Note: All cases of prolonged diarrhea (lasting several weeks) aggravate nutrient absorption, creating deficiencies as well as dehydration. Take extra vitamins and minerals for several weeks. Liquid forms are easier to assimilate, if you can get them.

Supplements to Heal the Intestinal Lining After *Chronic* Diarrhea

Rebuilding your intestinal lining and ecology prevents chronic problems down the road.

Take Several of the Following for One Month

- *Deglycyrrhizinated licorice* (DGL). Chew 1 or 2 380-mg tablets on empty stomach three or four times a day. This coats, soothes, and helps rejuvenate intestinal lining. Take twenty minutes before meals.
- *Glutamine.* 500-mg one to three times a day for positive "growth" effect on intestinal lining.
- *Vitamin A.* 5,000 IU once a day. (Do not take vitamin A if you are pregnant without consulting a physician.)
- *Zinc picolinate.* 30 mg once or twice a day and 2 mg copper at another time of day.
- *Vitamin B.* complex twice a day.
- *L. acidophilus* and *Saccharomyces boulardii.* 2 or 3 capsules two to four times a day.
- *Digestive enzymes.* (See chapter 19 to see if you may be helped by these and how much to take.)

Also consider trying these for chronic diarrhea:

Folic acid. 5 mg a day (large dosages reduce various diarrheas).

Oil of oregano. 1 capsule at meals and at bedtime. Emulsified oil of oregano has natural antibiotic, antiviral, and antiparasitic properties. It also inhibits friendly bacteria, so you need to consume probiotics several times a day at a different time from when you take this oil.

N-acetyl-D-glucosamine. 500 mg two to four times a day.

THE ACID SOLUTION

Sarah was healthy, young, athletic, and energetic, but she had been suffering with severe diarrhea for four years. She had seen many doctors who ultimately shook their heads. She didn't have fatigue, illness, or any other health problems, other than the fact that her rectum was constantly irritated. Something was wrong, but no one could diagnose the problem.

Her best friend was a nurse who heard me lecture at a relicensing seminar for nurses and Ph.D.s in public health. I mentioned that sometimes chronic diarrhea is a sign of inadequate stomach acid and she told Sarah, who started taking hydrochloric acid supplements. She began with one 8-grain capsule per meal and, when she got up to two per meal, within several days her diarrhea stopped. Even though I never met her, she sent me flowers.

Soothing Liquids for Diarrhea

Herbal Teas   Make a strong tea of slippery elm, peppermint, red raspberry, and 1/2 teaspoon cinnamon. Sip the tea throughout the day. If you don't have all these teas, use whichever one you have.

Other soothing herbs are chamomile, yarrow, and nettle.

Allantoin is an herbal extract that soothes the intestinal lining. Look for this on commercial labels of soothing GI products.

Vegetable Broth   Cut up whole unpeeled potatoes along with any vegetables you have, such as carrots, onions, and celery. Put in a pot of water and cook for two to four hours, then strain. Sip this healing broth, which is high in natural potassium, throughout the day.

Juice Soup   Steam carrots, broccoli, onion, and zucchini. Add garlic if you like. Blend and warm, and add seasoning to flavor.

Blended Fruit "Soothie"   Blend banana, yogurt, and 1 teaspoon of organic applesauce with adequate water to make a pleasant consistency. You may add cinnamon to taste. You can also add 1 teaspoon of a supplement if you want.

Diarrhea in Infants and Children

Infants up to 18 Months Old

Infants are so small that a relatively small amount of diarrhea and/or vomiting can quickly cause the loss of a major portion of their circulatory volume. This means they can dehydrate quickly, which can be fatal. *Call a doctor immediately* if your infant has had diarrhea for over two hours or appears listless, unresponsive, and inappropriately drowsy; develops dry mouth and tongue, glazed eyes, and loose skin; cries constantly; or if the fontanel (soft spot) at the front of the head seems too "sunk in" or depressed.

Avoid giving milk to your infant for 24 hours, even human milk. Instead, give generous amounts of rice water (see page 80) or commercially available electrolyte solutions for infants, such as Pedialyte. You can mix either of these with 1 teaspoon of *Bidifidus* (Natren has a product that has *Bifidobacterium infantus* in it), along with liquid vitamins and minerals for infants (give dosage recommended on the label).

The use of fiber-supplemented soy formula (Isomil DF) has been shown in studies to reduce acute diarrhea in infants six months of age and older. Ask your doctor before giving anything to your baby.

Children

Diarrhea in an otherwise healthy child (between the ages of one and four years old) is defined as having five or more watery or loose stools a day. Children can dehydrate rapidly. Call a doctor immediately if there is mucus or blood in their loose stools, if the rectal temperature is 102°F (38.9°C) or higher, or if your child seems lethargic or nonresponsive, doesn't want to eat, cries constantly or has had diarrhea for several hours. Ask your doctor about any of the recommendations in this section.

Most childhood diarrhea (acute gastroenteritis) is caused by viral infections or abusing fruit juices (see below). Viral infections can damage the lining of the small intestines and create lactose intolerance (inability to digest milk sugar), which can cause secondary diarrhea. *So avoid milk or milk products for at least two weeks during and after a strong bout of diarrhea.*

Give your child 6 to 8 glasses of fluid a day. Give 1 teaspoon or 2 capsules of a*cidophilus* on an empty stomach three or four times a day. Do not yell or create tension around any "accidents" (the inability to make it to the bathroom). This may aggravate the problem and create more psychological ones. Try 20 mgs of zinc a day for a week, multivitamins and minerals (liquid children's products), apple pectin or bananas mashed in applesauce, and chamomile tea sipped throughout the day.

Homeopathics are natural aids that are available at your health-food stores and helpful for childhood diarrhea. They are described in such books as *Homeopathic Medicine* by Trevor Smith, M.D., (Healing Arts Press, 1989) and *Everybody's Guide to Homeopathic Medicines* by Steven Cummings and Dana Ullman (Tarcher and St. Martin's Press, 1984).

Some of the most commonly used homeopathics for diarrhea in children are:

Pulsatilla, used especially if no two stools are alike, the diarrhea is worse in the evening, the child cries a lot and/or the diarrhea started after eating fatty or starchy foods.

Arsenicum album, used especially for severe diarrhea—if your child seems very ill, exhibiting chills, vomiting, diarrhea, and restlessness, if there is a lot of mucus, burning, and the stools are often green or pale.

Phosphoric acid and *podophyllum* are used more often in chronic cases.

When traveling or if there is an intestinal infection going around the school that causes diarrhea, *L. rhamnosus strain* GG (L-GG) has been shown to prevent diarrhea and to shorten its course once contracted, in children.

Child's Diarrhea and Fruit Juices

Chronic nonspecific diarrhea is a common problem in which diarrhea occurs in children six months through four-and-a-half years of age who have three or more loose stools a day *for at least three weeks*. This is very often caused by fruit juices, especially apple juice and pear nectar (they contain sorbitol or fructors in excess of glucose) and malabsorption of them is not uncommon. Take your child off juices or give 2/3 water, 1/3 grape juice, which is better tolerated. Over-consumption of juices has been linked with failure to thrive, cavities, obesity, and kidney stress in children.

Mind-Body Techniques

Reflex Points for Diarrhea

When doing reflex points for diarrhea, do not use a lot of pressure. Be gentle. Find the most tender spots on the digestive, colon, and rectum points of the feet. Hold these areas with your thumbs. Breathe gently into these areas and visualize the associated organs relaxing. With your nail, gently stimulate the tip of the large toe (an unconventional reflex point now found to be helpful for diarrhea). (See foot reflexology charts at the end of chapter 20.)

Soothing Exercises for Diarrhea

1. *Relax-a-Colon.* Lie on your back with a pillow under your knees. Put the palms of both hands on your abdomen. Breathe into your palms, visualizing your breath to be a golden light. Exhale this light directly from your palms into your abdomen. Attempt to "feel" the warmth of this light. Keep breathing until you feel your abdomen warm up. If you can't accomplish this, work with a hot water bottle placed on a towel on your abdomen. Be careful not to burn yourself. Only do this exercise for ten minutes.

2. *Baby Pose with Fists.* Sit on your heels on the floor. If this is too uncomfortable for you, sit on a chair. Make gentle fists with both hands. Place them on your abdomen under your rib cage. If you are on your heels, lean forward and touch your forehead as close to the floor as you can. If you are on a chair, lean your forehead toward or onto your knees, whichever is comfortable. Breathe

deeply at least ten times. This gives a gentle massage to your abdomen without a lot of motion. Come up. Sit still for a few moments. You can build up to doing this pose for 20 to 30 minutes. It is gentle and easy to do, but very effective.

Affirmations for Diarrhea

Sit or lie down quietly with the palms of both hands on your abdomen. Breathe deeply three times.

Relax, and while you inhale, say to yourself, *"I inhale peace."*

Exhale and say, *"I calm down."*

Inhale, *"Peace."*

Exhale, *"Calm down."*

After a while, when you feel gentle stillness, ask yourself, "Why am I having this problem?"

See what answers you can learn from yourself.

Also try the heating and cooling meditations and affirmations recommended in chapter 6 for heartburn.

9 *Keys to Overcoming Diverticular Disease*

When you are born, your intestinal tract is a smooth healthy tube with a muscular layer. During childhood, you might eat many meals at fast-food restaurants. As you grow up and try to take more charge of your health, you might think at first that switching to whole-wheat bread supplies all your fiber needs (wrong—this is a small part of the picture). Perhaps you start to eat salads once in a while, but you don't consume a variety of whole grains like brown rice, buckwheat, or millet, or seeds like flax, sunflower, pumpkin, and raw nuts. You think healthy eating is dining on macaroni, pasta, and a noncoarse whole-wheat bread. You overeat desserts, cookies, and candies, but you're pleased with yourself because you're taking a multiple vitamin/mineral.

All the while you are living on this low-fiber, high-sugar diet, changes are happening to your once-smooth intestinal tube. It develops little out-pouches of the muscular wall, which are small *hernias* in the muscular layer. These sacs are more likely to occur on your left side (descending and sigmoid colon), but can occur throughout your colon. Parts of the colon sag. Other parts contract, decreasing the diameter. You may look beautiful on the outside, but your colon is aging.

By age forty-five, 30 to 40 percent of an American's once-healthy colon is riddled with lumps, bumps, and constrictions. This is called *diverticular disease.* It increases in severity as we get older. It is estimated that more than three-fifths of people over the age of seventy have it. With the U.S. population living longer, diverticular disease is becoming an increasingly common problem.

How Diverticular Disease Develops

Eating the dangerous twins—*low-fiber foods and high-refined-sugar foods*—increases the pressure inside the colon. This increased pressure causes the weakened colonic wall to develop diverticular herniations.

Inflammation of the colonic wall around these diverticuli can cause isolated bouts of pain or chronic pain. Diverticuli can get infected (diverticulitis), which may cause attacks severe enough to require surgery. Or the sacs may harbor unfriendly bacteria, which inhibit digestion and create a toxic load on the body and the immune system.

The sigmoid—the lower S-shaped part of your colon—is the most frequently affected (90 percent of the time), because this is the narrowest segment of your colon. This portion develops the highest internal pressure when any portion of your colon starts to develop tension. If you eat a typical fast-food diet and don't exercise regularly, all these changes may be happening to you.

In one study, diverticular disease was consistently found more frequently in nonvegetarians (33 percent) than in vegetarians (12 percent). The vegetarians who did develop diverticular disease ate less cereal fiber than the vegetarians who did not get diverticular disease.

Genes play a role in diverticular disease, too. If one of your parents had it, you have a chance of getting it, and if both have it, you have a bigger chance.

What Happens When You Eat Doughnuts Often?

When you eat any food, like a doughnut, which is high in the dangerous twins, sugar and fat, while low in fiber:

Your stomach feels less full than if you ate higher-fiber foods.

You tend to overeat.

You crave high-sugar, low-fiber foods. (Once you start eating cookies, cakes, and pastries, it's hard to stop.)

These foods cause unequal pressures on the intestines, which causes normal motility to be disrupted, which in turn creates hernias—or diverticular disease.

Common Symptoms of Diverticuli

Some people don't have overt symptoms (at least for the first few decades). This is called *symptomless diverticular disease.*

Some people have frequent pain, even in the absence of evident inflammation. This is called *painful diverticular disease* or *spastic colon diverticulosis.* The pain is thought to be partially due to spasms of the colon.

Diverticular pain usually manifests as localized tenderness over the lower-left side. It also may show up as lower-left-side pain that feels as if there is a lump or mass. Diverticular pain may be intermittent and vary in intensity. Vague lower-left-sided abdominal pains with possible episodes of heightened pain (attacks) also suggest diverticulitis.

Abdominal distress after eating is common, and sometimes diverticuli can cause rectal bleeding (mild to severe).

People with histories of gallbladder disease, obesity, and heart disease, as well as people where parents had diverticuli (genetic predisposition), are at greater risk.

Eating Hints to Treat Diverticuli

- Eat one *whole grain* a day—whole cooked oat, millet, rice, buckwheat, rye, etc. Try eating whole grains for breakfast instead of cereal out of a box. Try whole grains with cooked vegetables on top as an accompaniment to your protein (meat, eggs, fish, tofu, beans, or tempeh) for dinner.
- Eat cooked *beans* several times a week.
- Eat lots of *vegetables* (try to have some raw, some cooked) not just as side dishes, but as main dishes, and consume moderate amounts of fruit.
- Have a *fiber cocktail* once a day (see chapter 2, page 25).
- Identify *food allergies,* which can aggravate diverticuli (see chapter 18).
- Do not eat refined sugar daily. Save it for a treat. It is not what you eat once in a while that "gets" you—it's what you eat most of the time that influences your health.
- Do not eat refined flours, such as refined rice, bread, pasta, cookies, bagels, and cakes on a daily basis.
- Cut out or reduce cow's-milk products.

Dairy Products and Diverticular Disease

A number of medical doctors reported in the *British Medical Journal* that when they took their patients with recurrent diverticulitis off milk, their symptoms disappeared. They questioned whether diverticular disease is becoming more common as Westerners consume more dairy products. Is this an allergy situation? Are the larger casein proteins harmful to the colonic walls? Is it the chemicals in the milk? Whatever it is, *if you have diverticular disease, you'll probably benefit by cutting down or eliminating cow's-milk products.*

Cow's-milk products are high in milk sugar (lactose). Sugar makes up about a third of the calories in milk. Milk sugar is a sugar source we often forget about. If you are eating many dairy products each day (cheese, milk, ice cream, and dairy products added to other foods) this is adding to your body's overall burden of sugar. Add a low-fiber diet and you have the *dangerous twins* again, and potential for developing a diverticuli problem.

Avoiding milk does not need to put you at risk for fragile bones. Dark-green leafy vegetables and raw seeds are high in calcium. These sources are actually more easily assimilated than the calcium in milk. Also, cheese is a very constipating food and constipation aggravates and contributes to diverticular disease.

Juices for Diverticular Disease

- Juice or blend carrots, cabbage, and beets.
- Blend pineapple juice and water with a few sprigs of parsley and/or mint.
- Juice or blend ginger, celery, carrots, and apples.
- Juice or blend garlic, tomatoes, carrots, and sweet green or red peppers.

Desserts for Diverticular Disease

- Blend cooked oats with soy milk and add applesauce to taste.
- Mix brown rice with thawed frozen berries and soy milk.
- Cut up fruit, such as pears and peaches, into little pieces. Add cinnamon and yogurt or cultured cottage cheese.

What to Do if You Have a Diverticular Attack

Eat lots of soft cereals. It is especially good to cook whole grains with twice as much water as usual. For example, cook 1 cup of brown rice in 4 cups water. Cook for two hours, twice as long as usual. Eat as is or add cut-up fruit or apple or berry sauces. This is very soothing to the colon.

Try blended soups. Steam cut-up carrots in water. When soft, put them in a blender with the water left at the bottom of the pot. Blend with a little butter.

Avoid whole seeds and nuts.

Drink fiber cocktails twice a day (see chapter 2).

Take 3 to 4 probiotics capsules two to four times a day for a week (see chapter 3).

Try several of these nutrients for one to three weeks:

- 1/4 cup of *liquid aloe* once or twice a day.
- 1 gram of *glutamine* twice a day.
- 5,000 IU of *vitamin A* daily.
- 400 IU of *vitamin E* daily.
- Several hundred mg of *bromelain* several times a day between meals.
- 1 B complex once a day.
- 2 tablets of *deglycyrrhizinated licorice (DGL)* chewed several times a day on an empty stomach 20 minutes before meals.

After an attack, determine whether you need digestive enzymes (see chapter 19), continue bromelain between meals twice a day (100 to 300 mgs), take 2 garlic capsules with meals, 1 to 2 grams of vitamin C, as well as the other nutrients mentioned above for one month. Consume probiotics daily in food or capsules. Take a fiber cocktail once a day on an ongoing basis. Drink chamomile, papaya, or peach teas. Celestial Seasonings "AM Detox" is a pleasant tea on rising and before bed. It is especially good steeped for a long time in combination with peach or peach detox teas. Herbs in capsules that are helpful for diverticular problems are cayenne, red chili, and yarrow.

Diverticulitis: Inflammation

Diverticulitis occurs when a diverticula becomes inflamed or infected. This can lead to serious trouble, such as blockage of your intestines or the bursting of a hole through your intestines. The hernias or sacs can fill up with pus and create complications (abscess and fistulas).

Extreme left-sided pain with fever, which may be accompanied by stiff muscles in your abdomen, may be diverticulitis, which is an emergency situation. Sometimes the pain can be down near the genitals, or on your right side, mimicking appendicitis. Sometimes the pain will get worse when urinating, suggesting that a ruptured diverticula has scarred your bladder. All these symptoms must be checked by a doctor.

Soft-tissue abdominal muscular or ovarian problems can mimic diverticular disease (see chapter 9). A doctor must rule these out.

Mind-Body Techniques

Reflex Points for Diverticular Disease

With the knuckles or thumb, start at the heel and work up the outside of the right foot, up to the middle, then across to the instep. Then work from the instep of the left foot across to the side of the foot and down to the heel. Work the center of these areas on both feet. Use the nail to stimulate both big toes (unconventional reflex points now found to be helpful for this condition).

Finish by working the original path up the right foot, across to the left foot, and down. Start and finish in this order. This helps relieve abdominal pain, gas, and distention, usually within ten to fifteen minutes. Finish with three deep breaths. Visualizing your breath helps to relax the intestines. (See reflexology charts at the end of chapter 20.)

Yogic Healing Exercise (Modified)

Sit comfortably on a chair. Hold your arms out at shoulder height. Take three deep breaths. Then, as slowly as possible, lift your arms so your hands touch above your head. With your hands together above your head, take three more breaths.

Now bring the palms down to your abdomen, below your navel. On the inhale, visualize your breath "collecting" in your palms. On the exhale, visualize your breath going from your palms into your intestines. Continue to breathe like this for at least several minutes. Then lean over and put your head toward or on your knees. Sit like this for several minutes. Get up slowly so as not to get dizzy.

Affirmation

Lie down. Place your hands on your abdomen. Take three deep breaths.

Inhale and say, "*I relax and heal my intestines.*"

Exhale and repeat, "*I relax and heal my intestines.*"

10 *Easy Prevention and Cure of Hemorrhoids*

Now we are getting to the bottom of things, so to speak. You have three cushions of tissue at the bottom of your anal canal that help keep your anal canal closed. They act as a gentle barrier to keep fecal material inside the body until the appropriate time. The importance of these three little tissues is indisputable.

Problems with these cushions of tissue are called *hemorrhoids* or *piles*.

These tissues can get inflamed, swell, become engorged with blood, rupture, and tear. They have a generous blood supply, so if damaged, they bleed easily and sometimes profusely. Just as varicose veins occur in the legs, varicose veins can occur in the anal area; that's what hemorrhoids are, and they can occur internally and externally.

Common Symptoms of Hemorrhoids

You can have one or several of these symptoms: rectal pain, rectal bleeding, protrusion of tissue, swollen tissues, fresh red blood on toilet paper, painful evacuation of stools, mucus discharge, and sensation of incomplete evacuation. These symptoms usually mean the hemorrhoids are internal.

Note: Rectal bleeding has to be checked by a doctor to rule out serious health problems such as ulcerative colitis, cancer, etc.

Hemorrhoids occur universally in adults and children. But this hardly means they are normal. Like other digestive problems, hemorrhoids are a sign of imbalance in diet and lifestyle. The good news is that often simple changes bring about simple healing.

THE CREATIVE ARTIST WITH A PROBLEM

Ron was a glassblower. He created beautiful pieces that sold all over the country. But he was troubled with severe rectal bleeding. His doctor ruled out cancer, diagnosed Ron's problem as hemorrhoids, and suggested surgery. Ron was mulling this over when a new customer walked into his studio. The man was a doctor. He and Ron got to talking. The doctor heard Ron's complaints and offered a trade. He would give Ron a free medical visit for one of Ron's pieces of art. Ron agreed.

The doctor first rechecked Ron and agreed the problem was severe hemorrhoids. He then asked Ron what he ate. Ron ate lots of whole-fiber foods, so he couldn't understand how this had happened to him.

The doctor said Ron's problem was that he needed more soluble fiber. He recommended that Ron take 2 teaspoons of psyllium husks in water twice a day followed by a large glass of plain water. That was it. Nothing else. In one week Ron's hemorrhoids went away. He kept up this simple program and they never returned.

Causes of Hemorrhoids

- *A sedentary lifestyle.* I know a number of health-minded people who eat excellently but don't exercise, and they are prone to hemorrhoids.
- *Eating fiber-deficient foods, too many sweets,* and drinking inadequate fluids.
- *Abdominal muscle strain* due to heavy or improper lifting, childbearing, and straining from constipation.
- *Overweight.*
- *Constipation overloads the colon.* The overloaded colon presses against the large veins of the pelvis, which makes the circulation to the genitals, anus, and legs sluggish (see chapter 7 on constipation).
- *Normal evacuation with harder consistency.* In other words, you don't have to be *severely* constipated. Too little exercise and inadequate fiber and fluids cause harder stools. Hard stools create straining to evacuate. This straining fills the hemorrhoidal cushion tissues with blood. The pressure builds in these cushion tissues, and they balloon out like small grapes or small plums and can rupture. The cushion tissues can break away from where they are attached to the anal sphincter muscle. This causes bleeding, protrusion of tissue, and pain.
- *Genetics.* The tendency to develop hemorrhoids can be passed on in families.

HEMORRHOIDS AND A COUCH POTATO

Al was very careful about what he ate. He shopped only at the health-food stores and he ate lots of high-fiber foods. He was astounded when he got hemorrhoids. His were protruding and painful and he couldn't walk—a severe case. His doctor said that he might need surgery. Al became desperate. He talked at length with the woman at the health-food store, who recommended nutrients, soluble fiber, and aspirin, yet even those didn't work. He finally talked to a friend who was a physical trainer. The friend told Al that lack of exercise was a cause of hemorrhoids, just like lack of fiber.

Al hated to exercise. He bragged about being a couch potato—a healthy couch potato. But Al didn't want surgery. So Al began to either swim or walk every morning. In two weeks his hemorrhoids improved; in three weeks they were gone. Al was amazed that diet wasn't enough, but he was glad he had figured out how to avoid surgery—even if it meant losing his couch potato status.

Tips for Hemorrhoids

Slant Board

Just as varicose veins are helped by putting the legs up higher than the heart, so are hemorrhoids helped by a slightly inverted position. You can use a slant board or lie on the floor and prop your buttocks and legs up on a bed or chair. The idea is to have your pelvis and intestines *upside down*, which gives them a rest. Relax five to ten minutes but not more than twenty. Get up slowly. Do not do this if you have eye or brain disorders.

Fiber keeps the stools smoother, which reduces pressure, and it moves food through you faster so it doesn't lose as much water. This prevents constipation, which keeps the circulation to your anal tissues healthier. Fiber also keeps you from overeating, which protects you from constipation. Try a fiber cocktail (see chapter 2, page 25) or eating a bran muffin on rising and before bed.

Drink plenty of fluids. Try the healing teas mentioned below. Chew food very thoroughly before swallowing, and eat slower.

Wear looser-fitting clothes.

Try sitz baths: Soak in a little warm water for 20 minutes daily or several times a day. Add mineral salts to the water if you like, especially the chemical-free ones found in health-food stores.

Have periods of rest with your legs and pelvis higher than your heart.

Natural Herbal and Homeopathic Treatments

Try one or two of the following for several days, and if they don't help try the others.

- One tablespoon of *flaxseed oil* once a day.
- If flaxseed oil doesn't help, consider *vitamin E* (400 IU) orally as well as using a 400-IU vitamin E capsule as a suppository at night before going to bed, for ten days. Be gentle. Don't insert roughly or too high up. If you don't have E available, use witch hazel, gently rubbed into tissues.
- *Bioflavonoids* (such as hesperidin and rutin). Take a bioflavonoid complex of 400 to 1,000 mg daily, for one month. Then reduce to several hundred milligrams a day. Also, eat buckwheat groats, which are very high in rutin. Juice organic citrus fruit, an excellent source of hesperidin.
- Add *vitamin B$_6$* to your diet: 100 mg twice a day until you get relief, then reduce to 50 mg once a day. The lack of this vitamin has been shown to contribute to hemorrhoids, and supplementation has been shown to help heal

them. Pregnant women often suffer with hemorrhoids, and one cause may be low levels of vitamin B$_6$.

- *Homeopathic aloe,* 30C taken as 5 pellets three times a day, or 12C taken as 5 pellets every hour until the problem starts to lessen, then reduce to three times a day until you are fine.
- There is a Chinese remedy called *Fargelin,* which is inexpensive and effective. Take as instructed on the bottle. However, some Chinese herbs have been found to have heavy metal contamination. Plum Flower brand certifies that their herbs have safe levels.
- Try homeopathics (oral and suppository).
- If you have *recurrent hemorrhoids,* take *liver decongestants* (milk thistle and/ or yellow dock, several capsules two or three times a day) for one month to reduce toxic liver burden.

Other Suggestions for Hemorrhoids

- Take 1/2 cup of aloe two or three times daily.
- Do an intestinal detoxification and rebuilding program (see chapter 20).
- Take 250 mg of magnesium three times daily. (Too much of this natural stool softener may cause mild diarrhea. If this occurs, cut the dosage back. Stools should normalize within the next day or two.)
- Take 1 tablespoon of chlorophyll two or three times daily.
- Try teas made from buckthorn bark and/or collinsonia root.

Morning Wake-Ups for Hemorrhoids

Breakfast on bran muffins or buckwheat groat cereal with fruit. Drink grapefruit, orange, and lemon juice mixed together. You can also blend with half a diced Granny Smith apple.

Note: Do not take grapefruit juice and the medication Seldane at the same time. Grapefruit juice (not other citrus juices) can inhibit an enzyme in the body that detoxifies this drug, resulting in adversely elevated levels.

Ultimate Morning Delight Cut up half a banana and half an apple and blend with one helping of Ultimate Meal, several almonds, and diluted organic apple juice or just plain water.

Carrot, Coconut, and Greens Juice carrots. Add a little liquid canned coconut juice (or juice fresh coconut meat, if you have it) and blend with a helping of greens, like spinach, or add a teaspoon of chlorophyll or green powder.

Pudding in a Drink Place cooked grain, such as brown rice, millet, quinoa, or oats (1 cup per person) in a blender with one teaspoon of organic currants and add soy milk to desired consistency. You may add fruit, such as apples or applesauce, peaches, berries, or pears.

Mind-Body Techniques

Reflex Points for Hemorrhoids

Sit comfortably. Use your knuckles to work deep into the bottoms and heels. It's difficult to get deep enough here, so use good pressure. Stimulate in little circles, several times, back and forth. If you find a very sore point, press deeper and hold until the pain in the sorest point seems to lessen.

Repeat for several minutes, morning and night, for one month.

Stand up. Walk around the house on your heels for 25 counts. Do this only if it does not strain your feet, knees, hips, or back. Relax. Repeat. This stimulates the anal reflex points. (See foot reflexology charts at the end of chapter 20.)

Healing Exercises for Hemorrhoids

1. *Joan's Exercise.* My friend Joan had such a large hemorrhoid she used to called it "the hemorrhoid about to take over Santa Fe." She successfully used this exercise, along with sitz baths, bran muffins, and homeopathics, to cure it.

   Put your hands on the back of a chair for support and have your legs gently bent, not locked. You are going to be exhaling rapidly with force 25 times so that, as you look down, you can see your diaphragm and abdomen go in and out. When you are done, sit down slowly to avoid getting dizzy. If this makes you dizzy, start with 10 times and build up to 25.
2. *Buttocks Lift.* Lie on your back on the floor. Bend your knees so your heels are by your buttocks. Squeeze your anus and gently lift your buttocks off the floor several inches, then lower down again. Repeat this 20 times.
3. *Hemorrhoidal Kegel Exercises.* This exercise is a squeezing motion done standing. Squeeze the rectum and your lower abdominal area up toward the navel. Hold these tissues in this upward clenched movement for several seconds and then release. Repeat 10 times. Build up to 50 times once or twice a day. This is good for treating as well as preventing recurrence of hemorrhoids. It is a combination of a modified Kegel exercise plus a variation on a yogic technique called *bandhas*.
4. *Yogic Healing Exercise.* Kneel on the ground. Bend over and place the top of your head on the floor with your hands by your ears, as though you were going to do a head stand—don't worry, you're not! Straighten your legs so that your bottom is in the air, your head is down, and your legs are apart, further than shoulder width. Or sit on a chair and put a pillow across your abdomen. Bend your head to your lap and do the exercise from this position.

   Relax your buttocks and anus. Get comfortable in this pose. Now, squeeze your anus as tightly as you can, as though you could draw it up to your belly button. Then relax. Repeat this 20 times.

   Come down or up slowly and relax.

Visualization and Affirmation

Sit or lie down quietly. Bring your awareness to your anal area. Tighten it as hard as you can for as long as possible, then release and relax it completely. Do this several times. Breathe deeply three times.

Imagine a ball of green light the size of a grapefruit sitting on top of your head. With each exhale, let this round, green light start to sink into your body. First, it fills up your head, face, and neck. Then, always on the exhale, it sinks down into your chest and into the rest of your body. Let this soothing color and sensation sink into your digestive tract and finally down into the rectum. Feel the light and coolness fill all the tissues.

When you have completed this visualization, with your focus on your anus, say:

On the inhale, *"Heal."*

On the exhale, *"Repair."*

Repeat for as long as comfortable. Relax for a short time before getting up.

11 *Natural Answers for Inflammatory Bowel Disease*

Inflammatory bowel disease is an overall name for a number of disorders whose symptoms overlap, making diagnosis confusing. The hallmark of inflammatory bowel problems is areas of *chronic inflammation* occurring at different sites in the gastrointestinal tract, anywhere from the mouth to the rectum.

What is inflammation? Inflammation means tissues are being irritated, injured, and destroyed. Inflammation can cause pain, heat, redness, swelling, and/or loss of normal functioning.

Inflammation in the intestinal tract means that at certain areas the intestinal lining is reacting to some kind of irritant. At these places the lining can have various degrees of the above five symptoms. The degree to which these five signs are present determines whether the inflammation is mild, moderate, or severe.

Inflammatory bowel disease is a term that includes conditions such as ulcerative colitis, Crohn's disease, and related conditions. Most inflammatory bowel diseases are usually chronic and debilitating, but I have found that the collection of tools I will share with you often greatly improves people's lives, reduces their pain, and quiets their conditions. They do not always make the illness go away, but in some cases there is complete healing. All inflammatory bowel conditions need to be monitored by professionals.

TEAM HEALING ULCERATIVE COLITIS

Tom and his wife were high school sweethearts who had been together for seventeen years. They were holding hands when they came in to see me, to discuss his lifelong battle with ulcerative colitis. Tom was hating the side effects of the cortisone and other drugs he was taking to keep his severe bowel disease only moderately under control. We put Tom on an elimination diet, avoiding food suspects in order to sleuth out allergies (see chapter 18 on allergies).

His worst allergic food turned out to be carrots. He had been drinking carrot juice daily, thinking it was a perfect food. He stopped eating carrots and other allergic foods and added nutrients, many of them in liquid form, and a daily green drink. He and his wife began sharing therapeutic foot massages, affirmations, and meditations every night. They focused on healing both their conditions (she wanted more energy and less PMS).

Tom was able to go off his medications within five weeks. He saw such a difference after stopping his allergy foods that he made a New Year's resolution. He promised to retest his food allergies once a year to make sure he didn't develop new ones and to keep avoiding the appropriate ones. Tom was a mentally healthy person who did what it took to heal himself.

What Type of Bowel Disease Might You Have?

Any part of the intestinal tract can get inflamed, and different names are given for each type of inflammation. *Colitis* is inflammation of the colon. *Enteritis* is inflammation of the small intestine. *Ileitis* is inflammation of the last part of the small intestine. *Proctitis* is inflammation of the rectum.

Colitis is the mildest form. Ulcerative colitis and Crohn's disease are more severe yet common forms of inflammatory bowel disease. The exact causes of inflammatory bowel disease are not known, but they may be partially autoimmune in nature, with the body attacking its own colonic tissue. Severe cases of inflammatory bowel disease usually develop complications such as extreme fatigue, nutrient deficiencies, arthritis, liver disease, kidney stones, colon cancer, and skin and eye disorders.

Colitis

Early colitis is characterized by abdominal pain, discomfort, cramps, colicky feelings, possible diarrhea, and the need to eliminate several times a day, sometimes with an urgency. Mild forms may have little or no symptoms.

Severe Colitis (Ulcerative Colitis)

This is a chronic condition of the colon and rectum, in which inflammation occurs along with ulcers. The hallmark *symptom* of ulcerative colitis is *blood and mucus* in the stools, along with abdominal pain and diarrhea. The stools can be loose or formed. Ulcerative colitis usually begins between the ages of twenty and forty with bloody diarrhea and severe abdominal pain attacks that vary in intensity and duration. There are cycles of attacks and healing. These cycles result in the narrowing of the intestinal tract, which can cause complications. Water and minerals are not well absorbed, so there is generally ill health, loss of appetite, weight loss with possible dehydration and anemia (low hemoglobin and low hematocrit), and general fatigue.

Crohn's Disease

Crohn's disease is a condition in which areas of inflammation occur anywhere along the intestinal tract. The areas most commonly affected are the last segment of the small intestine (ileum) and the colon. The inflamed areas extend through all the layers of the intestinal lining and may also involve the adjacent lymph nodes. *Symptoms* include chronic diarrhea, associated with abdominal pain usually on the right side (sometimes this is called the "right-sided disease"), bouts of severe fatigue, fever, weight loss, and right lower-abdominal fullness or mass. One third of people with this illness have complications with their rectum.

Many times the first symptom appears as an attack that mimics appendicitis or bowel obstruction. The first attack usually occurs around age twenty. First attacks may be several months or years apart. Sometimes one or two attacks occur and then never return. These cases are rare and are usually caused by an infection due to a live organism.

As Crohn's progresses, the intestinal functioning becomes more and more impaired. Abscesses, fistulas, pockets, and canals of infection can lead to and affect other organs. Untreated Crohn's disease can be serious.

Who Is at Risk?

The incidence of inflammatory bowel disease is increasing around the world.

Even though classic medical books often say there are no known or dietary causes of these illnesses, recent studies don't agree. Research, along with the steep rise of cases in the Western world, has implicated a number of risk factors. These factors work together, meaning that they are *additive*. Isolated, they are not directly linked to inflammatory bowel disease.

The risk factors implicated are the increased consumption of refined carbohydrates and sugars, non-nutritive additives, fatty foods, and dairy products; unbalanced eating habits; low-fiber diets; eating less fresh fruits and vegetables; and multiple food allergies. Many children with inflammatory bowel disease (about 70 percent) have lactose (milk sugar) intolerance, a genetic tendency for this illness, and altered intestinal bacteria. Since undetected parasite infections may cause and/or aggravate all types of inflammatory bowel disease, every person with this illness should have a comprehensive digestive and stool analysis or random stool tests taken three days in a row (see appendix B).

Possible causes of inflammatory bowel disease are infections due to various sources; damage to the intestinal wall from foreign molecules, or hypersensitive reactions to nonforeign molecules; undetected food allergies; nutrient deficiencies; and inflamed blood vessels. Standard treatments for inflammatory bowel disease are primarily cortisone-like drugs, anti-inflammatory drugs, antibiotics, and, in some cases, surgical removal of parts of the colon.

If *any* help can be gained by addressing nutritional and lifestyle factors, use of drugs and surgery and their side effects may be minimized or avoided.

How to Eat for Inflammatory Bowel Diseases (IBD)

Diet for All Types of Inflammatory Bowel Diseases

Eliminate sugar and refined carbohydrates: candies, sugar-sweetened drinks, chocolate, cakes, pies, ice cream, Jell-O, custard, cookies, and fruit juices, even those without added sugar.

Avoid stressor foods: caffeinated foods and beverages, processed oils, fried foods, colas, pastries, alcohol-refined grains, canned tuna, candies, sugared drinks, and other processed foods (see chapter 1).

Identify and avoid food allergies (see chapter 18) and try to rotate remaining food. A big culprit is dairy products (cow's milk products).

Avoid: undiluted fruit juices, excessive fruit or natural sugars, and overeating.

Drink 2 glasses of diluted fresh vegetable juice a day with 1 tsp green powder or liquid per day.

Go off birth-control pills, as these can contribute to IBD.

Improve your diet in this way for two weeks before adding supplements.

Be very careful to chew food well, sit in a relaxed, stressless atmosphere while eating, and consider giving thanks and doing affirmations given at the end of this chapter before and after meals (also see Mindful Hints in chapter 4).

Six Optimal Juices and Foods for IBD

Bowel Nourisher   Juice a slice of raw potato, broccoli, celery, cabbage, Granny Smith apple, and carrot.

Bowel Strengthener   Juice garlic, lemon, apple, ginger, and carrot.

Green Drink   Place parsley, spinach, four to five leaves of romaine lettuce, and pineapple juice in a blender. Blend and chew well.

Soy Almond Combo   Mix water, 1 serving of soy protein powder, half an apple, several almonds, and water. Blend well. Optimal: add 1/2 tsp of freshly ground flaxseeds.

GI-Friendly Drink   Blend soy yogurt with half a banana, almonds, and a little diluted juice.

Aloe Smoothie   Blend 1/3 cup of aloe vera juice with water and half an apple.

Herb Tea   Make tea from Pau D'Arco, valerian, mullein, and marshmallow. Add 1 teaspoon of chlorophyll, and unprocessed honey to taste. Sip throughout the day.

Healing Foods for Mild to Moderate Colitis

Adhere to this regime for approximately six weeks.

- *Eat three different vegetables* a day, all different colors, and one fruit, but no more than one piece of fruit a day for the first two weeks.
- *Eat a varied diet.* Rotate your foods as much as possible.
- *Do not eat several hours before bedtime.*
- Cut out dairy products for at least one month.
- Add *supplements* the third week.

Supplements for Mild to Moderate Colitis

Glutamine. 500 mg three times a day.
Vitamin A. 5,000 IU once a day.
Multiple vitamin/mineral.
Zinc picolinate. 30 mg once a day (balance with 2 mg of copper).
Probiotics. Such as *L. acidophilus*, 2 twice a day.
Bioflavonoids. 500 mg twice a day between meals for one month.
Healing herbs. 2 to 3 enterically coated peppermint oil capsules thirty minutes before meals, or 1/3 cup aloe vera once or twice a day, or 1/2 teaspoon of turmeric mixed with unprocessed honey once or twice a day.

Healing Foods for Severe Bowel Disease

Adhere to this regime strictly for at least three months.

- *Avoid sugar.* Eliminate all sugar products. You can have several tablespoons of fruit juice added to water. If you do cheat, eat the sugary foods along with other foods containing fiber or protein. The point is that you want to avoid the undiluted irritating effect of sugar against the intestinal lining.

    Studies in the United States and Israel have linked higher sugar consumption in the diet to people with Crohn's disease. Some studies showed that people with Crohn's disease consumed 90 percent of their carbohydrates as pure refined sugar products. Zinc is necessary to taste sweetness and saltiness. Zinc deficiency may cause the desire to eat more sweets. It is difficult to know if eating more sugar is a cause or a result of Crohn's.

- *Strictly avoid all dairy products.* The elimination of dairy products often greatly reduces spasms in the muscular wall of the intestine, and bloody diarrhea.
- *Avoid raw fruits and vegetables when bowels are loose.* Reintroduce these foods when the bowel movements are solid for more than three days. Until then, lightly steam or stir-fry your food. Eliminate all processed oils. Use mainly cold-pressed olive oil from organic sources when possible.
- *Identify food and inhalant allergies.* Numerous studies correlate ulcerative colitis with food allergies. Dairy products are the most common food offenders. Others may include wheat, corn, eggs, citrus fruits, coffee, tea, alcohol, sugar, and numerous food additives (see chapter 18).
- *Avoid chemicals and hydrogenated oils.*
- *Foods to focus on:* fish, lightly steamed greens, vegetables, potatoes, yams, squashes, legumes, seed and nut milks, eggs (if you are not allergic to them), some fruits (if stools don't get loose), lots of diluted fresh (not pasteurized) juices and green drinks, corn, quinoa, millet, brown rice, amaranth, and kamut grains.
- You *must eliminate* all alcoholic beverages, tomatoes and tomato-based products, canned tuna, and all saltwater fish (mercury has been shown by German researchers to be a factor in irritating the bowel).
- Avoid ice-cold drinks and drinking too many liquids with solid meals. Eat smaller, more frequent meals. Rotate foods as much as possible; for example, eat the same foods every two or three days instead of daily.
- Avoid yeasty foods, like bakery products.
- A study in the Scandinavian *Journal of Gastroenterology* showed that Crohn's disease activity was greatly reduced by eating a low-yeast diet (exclude vinegar, alcohol, breads, malted cereals, B vitamins from yeast sources, and refined sugars and flavors). Circulating antibodies to bakers' and brewers' yeast have been found in many Crohn's patients.

Supplements for Ulcerative Colitis (UC)

Add one new supplement a day—go slowly.
Don't take pancreatic enzymes.
L. acidophilus +/0 Bifidus. 3 or 4 capsules three or four times a day to enhance the production of butyrate, a short-chain fatty acid that healthfully "feeds" the colon.
Fish oil. Up to 10 capsules a day in divided dosages (if you have discomfort from the fish oil, take one capsule a day and slowly add one more at a time).
Vitamin A. Work with a doctor to determine dosage. Start at higher dosages and reduce as you get better.
Zinc picolinate. 30 mg twice a day (balance with 2 mg of copper).
Buffered Vitamin C. 1 gram twice a day.

Stomach acid supplements if there is a deficiency (see chapter 19).

PABA. Dr. Wright has observed that PABA (4 grams a day) is very helpful for ulcerative colitis, as it is very similar to the sulfasalazine molecule, a drug often prescribed for this condition. *PABA cannot be taken with sulfasala-zine or any sulfonamide drug, as it interferes with its action—so take one or the other.*

Folic acid. 400 mcg daily. Two well-designed studies have shown that folate may protect against UC patients developing cancer.

Aids for Ulcerative Colitis

Butyrate Enemas

A variety of studies have shown that a key nutrient for the cells that line the colon is *butyrate*, a short-chain fatty acid. Butyrate is formed in the colon by bacterial fermentation. Colon cells use butyrate the way we use food, for fuel and energy. People suffering with left-sided ulcerative colitis have been found to have inadequate levels of butyrate in their stool. A study in the *American Journal of Gastroenterology* (1994:89;179–183) discussed ten ulcerative colitis patients who had not responded to conventional therapies. These patients were given enemas that contained butyrate nightly for six weeks. Six of the ten patients improved. Four improved completely. Butyrate enemas are available by prescription; administer only under a doctor's supervision. Remember, taking oral *acidophilus* increases natural butyrate production in your gut.

Benefits of Fish Oil

Several studies have identified a benefit in taking fish-oil dietary supplements for ulcerative colitis. Fish oil contains omega 3 fatty acids. These fatty acids help reduce inflammation and excessive permeability that can occur in the colon and rectum of people with ulcerative colitis.

One study of ulcerative colitis patients showed that fish-oil therapy improved symptoms by 50 percent (although the tissue changes that occur with this condition were not improved). Some people were able to reduce or go off their medication.

In a study of 42 patients, published in *The American Journal of Gastroenterology* (Vol. 87, 1992), it was found that drugs could be reduced or eliminated in 72 percent of the cases while the patient was taking the equivalent of 10 capsules of fish oil a day. It was concluded that fish-oil supplementation improved symptoms in active mild to moderate cases of ulcerative colitis. Results have not been as clear-cut in people with Crohn's.

Nutrients and Crohn's Disease

Add one new supplement a day. Go slowly. *Don't take pancreatic enzymes or fiber supplements.* Use only as many of the following factors as you can comfortably handle.

Supplements for Crohn's Disease

Liquid multiple vitamin/mineral.

Zinc picolinate. 30 mg twice a day (balance with 2 mg of copper).

Vitamin A. Work with a doctor and start at higher dosages, then reduce when improved.

Fish-oil concentrate. 6 to 12 capsules a day.

Vitamin E. 800 IU once a day (keeps vitamin A levels higher and heals colon).

Folic acid. 1 to 10 mg a day.

Antioxidant formula. 1 capsule twice a day.

Probiotics. 2 to 4 capsules two to four times a day (*L. acidophilus* and *bifidus* enhance production of butyrate, which has a helpful immuno-suppressive action on the intestinal tract).

Glutamine: 1,000 mg three times a day for one month, then reduce to 500 mg once a day.

Buffered vitamin C. 500 mg two to four times a day. Build up very slowly over one or two months. Cut back if this causes loose stools and proceed slowly.

B complex (yeast-free). Once a day.

Calcium. 400 to 800 mg taken with meals. (reduced bone density can occur in Crohn's).

More Options to Consider

- *Sialex* is a unique product for inflammatory bowel conditions, as it contains sialic acid derived from bovine mucin. Take 3 or 4 capsules with each meal. In severe cases, take up to 8 capsules per meal, and when you improve, reduce the quantity until you are stable with improvement at 3 or 4 per meal.
- *Vitamin B_1 (yeast-free).* 100 mg once a day.
- *Vitamin B_{12}*, 1,000 mcg sublingually or intramuscularly, once a week.
- *Oxygenating formulas.* Aerobic 07 or Dioxychlor (see appendix B), 20 drops in a glass of water three times a day.
- *N-acetyl cysteine.* 100 to 300 mg capsule twice a day for one month to assist liver in detoxifying the toxic load that can leak across a damaged intestinal lining.
- *Soothing enemas* (see below).

Zinc

Numerous studies demonstrate that Crohn's sufferers have low-zinc tissue levels, attributed to a wide number of causes, from inflammation to increased need due to excessive loss. Many studies show that giving zinc to Crohn's patients (often the sole mode of therapy) may improve a significant number of the above problems, and, in rare cases, the Crohn's disease itself. Zinc is classically known to be a nutrient-promoting tissue healer.

Vitamin A

Vitamin A deficiency has been found in patients with active Crohn's disease. Vitamin A may be an essential nutrient in improving Crohn's. In the medical journal *The Lancet* (April 5, 1980), doctors discussed a thirty-one-year-old woman who was affected with this disease. She had part of her colon removed, but still had diarrhea twice a day. She was put on a high dose of vitamins A and E and within two weeks her bowel function returned to normal. They took her off and on the vitamins to figure out if it was the E or A that was helping her. It was the vitamin A. She was maintained on 100,000 units a day, even though her blood levels of vitamin A showed that she wasn't deficient in that vitamin.

After further study, the researchers figured out that vitamin A healed intestinal permeability. It stopped the *leaky gut* (the excessively permeable gut) associated with this illness. Also, low zinc levels found in many Crohn's sufferers may contribute to low levels of vitamin A, as zinc is needed to help absorb vitamin A.

Vitamin A appears to protect the barrier function of the intestinal tract in Crohn's and it stimulates healing and normalization of the colonic cells in ulcerative colitis patients. However, do not go over the RDA dosage of vitamin A (5000 mg daily) without a doctor's supervision.

Antioxidants

Tissue injury in Crohn's patients is partially due to oxidative (free radicals generated from the body's use of oxygen) damages to the intestinal wall, along with poor defense mechanisms in the intestinal wall to withstand this damage. It is conceivable that antioxidants would be helpful, and a number of studies support this viewpoint.

DHEA

Low levels of DHEA (an adrenal hormone) are often found in people with inflammatory bowel disease. Dr. Davis Larson at the Tahoma Clinic has noted that improving levels of DHEA (through low-dose supplementation) is often associated with improvement in ulcerative colitis symptoms.

Ask your doctor to run a blood test for DHEA. Inflammatory bowel disease is a family of autoimmune problems, and low levels of DHEA may aggravate this.

Soothing Enema

These are soothing, and decrease bleeding, irritation, and mucus in some individuals. Many of my patients felt this helped them to *get off* and *stay off* steroids. *Do this only with a doctor's supervision.*

Fill the enema bag with 1/3 cup of slightly warm (do not burn yourself) organic olive oil and 2 tablespoons of nonsugared soy-based liquid *acidophilus*. Pierce a 5,000-mg capsule of vitamin A and empty it into the mixture. You can also prepare an enema with just the olive oil. Optional: Add 1/4 cup of valerian tea or butyrate solution.

Mix all the ingredients and pour into a handheld small enema bulb. Gently squeeze into your rectum. Retain for as long as possible. This helps to ease the pain and enhances healing.

Improvement from Inflammatory Bowel Diseases

As your health improves, cut the supplements down and try to maintain as optimal a diet as possible, eating a wide variety of fresh foods and rotating them. According to Drs. Wright, Gaby, and Abram Ber, if a therapeutic program can be used to get people into remission, maintenance with a modified program can help prevent relapse.

If you are not improving, discuss the following points with your doctor and read *Breaking the Vicious Cycle* by Elaine Gotschall (Kirkton Press, 1994).

- *Test for parasites, bacteria, protozoa, helminthic, mold, and fungal infections, inhalant as well as food allergies.* All of these can contribute to inflammatory conditions of the bowel. Some cases of inflammatory bowel disease are greatly improved by identification and eradication of harmful organisms. The most common culprits are *e. coli*, *Staphylococcus*, and *Clostridium difficile* toxin. If you can't get tested, or if tests do not identify a harmful organism, consider going on a parasite or yeast program anyway for one month and see if you feel better (see chapters 15 and 16). Base your program on your symptoms, not only on laboratory results, which are not always accurate.
- *Test for excess or low stomach acid.*
- *Test for environmental allergies.* Seasonal flare-ups suggest an environmental allergy component.
- *Measles virus* has been associated with recurrences. (Olive-leaf extract may be helpful in viral problems).

Increased Risk for Thrombosis

Patients with either ulcerative colitis or Crohn's disease are known to be at an increased risk for blood clots, which frequently cause obstruction. Have your doctor test your *homocysteine levels.* If they are high, take folic acid, B_{12} and B_6, which have been shown to decrease this factor that increases the risk of thrombosis. One study showed that the level could be decreased within one month.

Mind-Body Techniques

Abdomen Massage

Mix 5 to 15 drops of rosemary oil into 1/4 cup of castor oil and 1/4 cup of olive oil. Warm this up and massage into the abdomen several nights a week before going to bed for a month.

Reflex Points for Inflammatory Bowel Disease

Sit comfortably. Relax. Hold your thumbs in the center of each foot. Slowly press deeper, gently stimulating your intestines. Hold for one minute.

Rub the entire middle of one foot, looking for the sorest points or feeling for little granules. Hold the sorest points until they hurt less. Work out any nodules you can feel under the skin by deep rubbing. Then do the toe tips and upper outside of the foot. Gently stimulate the tips of the toes with your fingernails, in small inching motions. Be gentle. Repeat on the other foot. See reflexology charts on pages 216–218.

Finish by holding both feet with your thumbs in the center of each. Inhale in and say to yourself, *"I inhale peace and health."*

Exhale and say, *"I give thanks for this peace and health."*

Do nightly for one month.

Affirmations

Healing Affirmation Before Meals (get in the habit of doing this all the time):

Sit in front of your food. Relax. Let your muscles go soft over the bones. Sigh out loud three times. Inhale and visualize drawing the breath into your intestines. Breath three times *into* your intestines.

Inhale and say, *"Relax."*

Exhale and say, *"Relax."*

Inhale, *"I accept this food perfectly."*

Exhale, *"I accept this food perfectly."*

Meditations

Do once a day for one month and then once to several times a week as you improve.

Abdominal Meditation #1 (music). Sit in a comfortable position. Hold your left palm over your abdomen, place your right palm over the left. Put on one of your favorite songs. Have the stereo set so the song keeps repeating itself. Let the music "collect" in your hands. Feel the music go from your hands into your abdomen. Feel the music fill up your abdomen. Sit there, letting your hands be a conduit for good feelings moving into your abdomen. Do this for as long as you like.

Abdominal Meditation #2 (warming). Put some castor oil on a piece of flannel or a washcloth. Take your shoes off. Lie on the floor on your back. Put your legs up on the seat of a chair. Place the castor oil side of the cloth on the bare skin of your abdomen, place plastic wrap over it, then put a hot water bottle on top. Be careful not to burn yourself.

Inhale. In your mind's eye, see gold light coming into your right palm and the sole of your right foot. See the gold light coming down your arm and up your leg, meeting in the center of your body, effusing your abdomen with healing golden light.

As you exhale, see your toxic darker energy leave your left side, down your arm and leg, out your palm and the sole of your foot. Continue this imagery as long as you like.

Exercise

Do once a day for one month.

Stand up. Roll your abdomen and pelvis around in circles, first to the right, then to the left. Do a circle in each direction ten times. While you are moving, *gently* percuss or "lightly tap" your abdomen with lightly closed fists. (Where you percuss, your body sends energy.) Do not *hit* yourself or tap too hard.

Transforming Emotions

Keep a weekly chart noting your emotions and your attacks. See if you notice any repeating patterns. Do your emotions relate to bouts of intestinal pain or problems?

Let's say you notice that whenever you feel *frustrated* (waiting in line, in traffic, with your children, etc.), several hours later you have an attack. So the idea is to transform your experience of frustration. How?

Be on the lookout for when you feel frustrated. When you start to feel frustration, think, "Now I have a chance to heal myself." Actively replace the thoughts of frustration with opposite thoughts, such as being thankful for something in your life. Replacing "destructive" thoughts with positive ones is an active part of healing. (This does not mean the destructive thoughts got you ill.)

12 *New Treatments for Peptic Ulcer and Inflamed Stomach*

Four members of one Dutch family walked into the Academic Medical Center in Amsterdam. They all had ulcers, but the unique thing was that they all had developed their ulcers at exactly the same time. Family members were tested and eight relatives were found to be infected with the same unfriendly bacteria. This is an example of ulcers being caused by a contagious "bug."

In 1959, a thirty-nine-year-old man who had had a duodenal ulcer for ten years went to see Dr. Breneman, an allergist. This problem patient had done all the conventional treatments and none of them had worked. He suffered with frequent hemorrhages because of his ulcer, and this caused severe fatigue. He had no history of allergies. Since there was nothing to lose, as nothing else had helped, Dr. Breneman placed this man on a food-elimination diet to see if he had food allergies. In three days, the man's ulcer symptoms stopped. He was found to be allergic to milk, wheat, and pork. The man stayed off these foods, healed his ulcer, saved his stomach (which the doctors had wanted to remove), and went on to live a healthful life. Dr. Breneman went on to write *Basics of Food Allergy.*

John owned a vitamin company. He worked too hard, drank too much, and frequently overate fast meals on the run. He developed an ulcer. Medication healed it, but when John stopped the medication, his ulcer came back and his digestion was worse than before. One of John's employees noticed him popping antacids by the water cooler. The worker said, "I've heard that some ulcers are caused by inadequate zinc. Look, you have white spots on your fingernails, which can be a sign of zinc deficiency. And a licorice extract is supposed to help, too." So John tried them both. He was pleasantly shocked when some of his own products, along with added fiber, helped heal his ulcer and kept it from returning.

These examples demonstrate that a variety of causes can reduce the ability of the stomach tissues to resist erosive damage. This new appreciation for multiple causes of ulcers gives rise to new treatments.

How to Recognize an Ulcer

In the United States, one out of every sixteen people develops ulcers. Men are more prone to ulcers than are women, and people with type O blood are more at risk. Also, if someone in your family has ulcers or gastritis, you are at greater risk of getting ulcers.

An *ulcer* is a craterlike area of damaged, inflamed, or dead tissue occurring in the mucous and muscular layer of whatever part of the intestinal tract is affected. In the stomach, ulcers occur with some degree of inflammation. However, stomach inflammation can occur without ulcers. This is called *gastritis*.

Peptic means related to the stomach and its juices. *Peptic ulcer*, however, does not refer only to a stomach ulcer. It is an umbrella term referring to *all* ulcers occurring within three areas of the upper digestive tract:

- the esophagus (the tube from the mouth to the stomach)
- the stomach itself (gastric area)
- and the duodenum (the stretch of small intestine leading away from the stomach).

The term *peptic ulcer* can refer to esophageal ulcers, stomach ulcers, or duodenal ulcers.

What Does It Feel Like to Have an Ulcer?

There are *common* and *uncommon* symptoms of ulcers.

Common symptoms of most ulcers include: Pain or aching, usually under the breastbone or upper abdomen area—the epigastric region. This pain can be burning, soreness, gnawing, sometimes an unexplained upper back pain (which actually is *referred* pain from an unknown ulcer), hunger pains that don't go away, or a chronic "empty feeling." The pain may be constant or it may come and go. It may vary from mild to moderate to severe, and is usually relieved by antacids or milk.

Specific ulcers can cause various types of uncommon pain:

Esophageal ulcer. Pain or burning over the breastbone area occurs more often during or after swallowing and occurs more frequently when lying down.

Stomach ulcer. Eating usually causes pain. Also bloating after eating, nausea, vomiting, and an unexplained feeling of being uncomfortably "full."

Duodenal ulcer. Pain over stomach area has consistent pattern: no pain on arising, then it appears by midmorning. Pain can be relieved by food but will reappear two to three hours after meals, frequently waking you up out of a sound sleep at 1:00 or 2:00 A.M. The pain may recur one or more times a day for several weeks and then may go away for months or several years without any treatment. Usually within two years, pain reoccurs. Recurrences are more common in transitional seasons (spring and fall) and during stressful and emotional life events.

Some people may not have any of the signals listed above until a complication occurs. Children may have very different symptoms. Elderly people may be unaware of problems until they have lost sufficient blood from bleeding ulcers to cause light-headedness on standing, shaking, fatigue, pale gums, white skin, and anemia.

Note: Any unexplained, ongoing anemia should be checked to see if an ulcer is causing it.

How to Know if You Have an Ulcer

Symptoms usually alert you. However, only 50 percent of people who have an ulcer get symptoms. The suspicion of an ulcer *must* be confirmed by a test because stomach cancer may have symptoms that mimic stomach ulcers, and you need to know what you are dealing with.

Get an endoscopic exam—visual inspection with a tool called an endoscope. However, this test can miss about 10 percent of gastric ulcers. Get X rays with barium studies, and blood tests for an ulcer bug.

Immediate Pain Relief from an Ulcer or Inflammation of Stomach

Take an antacid. Why suffer? If you don't have antacids on hand, try 1/4 teaspoon of baking soda in water. Antacids are great for blocking an acute episode, but do make a point of working your way into natural treatment and management as soon as possible. Ulcers take six to eight weeks to heal, depending on their severity, so consider that when using substances for immediate pain relief.

Why It Is Not Healthy to Keep Popping Antacids

Antacids, in the long run, don't work as well as supplements. A study published in *Surgical Gynecology and Obstetrics* (Feb:158, 1984) addressed this issue. Stressed rats usually develop ulcers. The authors (K. P. Lally and his colleagues) stressed 146 rats by depriving them of food and movement. They then compared the effectiveness of various nutritional supplements versus antacids in preventing ulcers. They concluded: "While the antacids were better than no treatment, they were significantly worse than any nutritional supplement."

Antacids can cause other serious health problems. Studies demonstrate that the aluminum present in many antacids is absorbed into the bones and brain where it may respectively promote osteoporosis and Alzheimer's disease. Fourteen women who used antacids for a year or more had significant bone loss because antacids block the absorption of phosphorus and stomach acid, which affect bones. This also shows that antacids are not a great way to get our calcium!

Other Options

- Take one large glass of water with 2 tablespoons of *aloe vera juice.* If you don't have aloe vera juice, try 2 tablespoons of *liquid chlorophyll,* and if you have only the water, just use that by itself. Water dilutes the acid in your stomach and moves it through.
- Chew 2 380-mg tablets of *deglycyrrhizinated licorice* (DGL) three to four times a day on an empty stomach.
- Stop eating your regular diet. For several days drink only fresh juices or eat steamed vegetables with whole grains. Drink fiber cocktails: Stir 2 teaspoons of *psyllium* into water and drink two to three times a day. Follow with a large glass of water with several teaspoons of aloe vera juice added. This is very soothing. Be very careful about eating habits while healing. Eliminate coffee, tea, colas, fried foods, refined sugars, refined carbohydrates, alcohol, and tobacco; identify and eliminate food allergies.
- Get a home *hemoccult* test kit from your local pharmacy, for testing blood in your stool. Once you've been diagnosed with ulcers, you should know if bleeding is occurring. Dark, blackish stools mean macrobleeding is occurring, but microbleeding, which isn't seen, can show up on this test. If bleeding is present your doctor *must* monitor your progress.
- Stop taking aspirin or nonsteroidal anti-inflammatory drugs. These medications irritate ulcers and promote bleeding.

Determining the Cause of Your Ulcer

Infection with an ulcer-causing bug, excessive use of aspirin and anti-inflammatory medication, nutrient and antioxidant deficiencies, emotional stress stimulating the production of excess stomach acid, food allergies, and low-fiber and high-refined-sugar diets are all potential causes or aggravating factors involved in ulcers.

Stress-Acid Theory

Generations of medical doctors have been taught that chronic stress releases stress hormones that cause the stomach to overproduce stomach acid—and this causes ulcers. But we now know that many people who have high levels of acid never get ulcers, and most people with ulcers have normal or even low amounts of acid. Yet, this theory still thrives, largely for commercial reasons. Pharmaceuticals, called histamine 2-receptor blockers (H2-receptor blockers), were introduced in the 1970s based on this high-acid theory. These drugs are effective. *But when an ulcer patient stops taking this medication, the ulcer usually returns.* To stay symptom-free, ulcer sufferers often have to be maintained on these drugs for years.

Because 5 to 10 percent of the world's population have either gastritis or ulcers at some time in their lives, these drugs have traditionally sold like wildfire. According to *Scientific American* (February 1996), "Major drug companies felt little incentive to explore or promote alternative models of peptic ulcer disease." This kept the acid-ulcer theory at the top of the list for a long time even though many ulcers have other causes.

Local Irritation Theory

Chronic use of aspirin, even enterically coated aspirin, and nonsteroid anti-inflammatory drugs (NSAIDs) are common causes of ulcers. Bleeding and irritation of the gastrointestinal tract can occur when more than 10 mg of aspirin are taken on a regular daily basis. This bleeding does not always show as black in your stools, which means you may not be aware that these drugs are causing irritation and bleeding. Sometimes bleeding ulcers occur as much as a month after rounds of aspirins or NSAIDs were taken.

Smoking decreases tissue levels of vitamins C and A. Both these vitamins protect against ulcer formation. Smokers (as well as people with chronic abdominal pain) often tend to eat less fruits and vegetables, which have higher levels of vitamins A and C. So smokers get a double deficiency whammy.

Moderate and excessive alcohol ingestion may irritate the stomach lining, as well as use up vital protective nutrients or be associated with a nutrient-poor diet.

Foods that stimulate the highest production of stomach acid and are therefore most likely to cause irritation are protein foods like meats and beverages like milk, beer, and wine. Thus, excessive consumption of these foods may contribute to ulcer formation.

Refined foods (low in fiber) can indirectly contribute to irritation. Refined flour products, such as white bread, white rice, and white pasta, can increase the risk of ulcers. The fiber in whole grains "buffers" your stomach lining from acid. Refined grains don't have this protective food-buffering effect because they don't have enough fiber.

An article in *The Lancet* on the protective use of dietary fiber in ulcer disease reports that 73 people who had just healed from duodenal ulcers were put on diets—half on a high-fiber diet and half on a low-fiber diet—for six months. Eighty percent of those on the low-fiber diet had recurrence of their ulcers. Forty-five percent on the high-fiber diet experienced recurrence. Smokers had a higher ulcer recurrence rate than did nonsmokers. It appears that a diet rich in fiber protects against duodenal ulcer.

Studies throughout the world correlate high ulcer incidence with national diets high in refined carbohydrates (low-fiber) and poor in nutrients.

Sugar Theory

A fascinating study was discussed by Dr. John Yudkin in the *British Medical Journal.* He was originally studying obese patients, but he noticed that people who were put on diets low in sugar had less heartburn. So he put seven healthy men on a diet high in sugar and low in whole grains and studied their stomach juices. After only two weeks on the high-sugar diet, stomach acid and pepsin activity increased by 20 percent. In other words, *diets high in refined sugar may increase stomach acidity above normal levels.* Eating refined sugars also changes fatty acid balance, which worsens ulcers.

Food-Allergies Theory

Dr. Jacob Siegel, an allergist, wrote that some stomach ulcers are allergic reactions to foods—in the lining of the stomach. Allergic patients release a lot of histamine, and ulcers can be caused by histamine. Food allergies can initiate histamine release and thus cause ulcer formation. Dairy products are the most common food allergen.

Nutrient and Antioxidant Deficient Theory

Specific nutrients and anti-oxidants *defend* the stomach lining from irritation and possibly from harmful bugs. Inadequate levels of zinc; vitamins A, C, and B_6; and possibly glutamine may contribute to ulcers. Supplementing these nutrients may help heal ulcers and prevent recurrences.

Why haven't you heard about these other causes of ulcers? Because medicine falls into patterns of philosophy and treatment. It often takes years, even in the face of valid information, to change an established mode of thought. Just because medicine has always treated an illness one way, or operated on the assumption that a disease is caused by certain factors, doesn't mean that's how it really is.

The Newest Theory of Ulcers: Bugs

Infection with a *bug*, a bacteria, is now a popular theory for what causes about *half* of peptic ulcers and stomach inflammation (gastritis). Perhaps over time, research will show that first other problems need to exist before infections by this bug can take hold and that the bug theory is not as clear as it appears to be. This is a controversial area and more research is needed.

The name of this bug is *Helicobacter pylori, H. pylori* for short. First, infection causes inflammation of the stomach. If the infection continues, it can lead to ulcers and possibly several forms of stomach cancer.

Most importantly, this organism can be easily identified and treated. Treatment lowers the chance of ulcer recurrence as well as the risk of gastritis and stomach cancer. Before discovering *H. pylori,* gastritis used to be considered a normal phenomenon of getting older and was called the "aging stomach." Now that *H. pylori* is known, gastritis can often be helped.

Many people are infected with *H. pylori.* Jay Hoofnagel, director of Digestive Diseases and Nutrition at the National Institute of Diabetes, Digestive and Kidney Disease Center, said, "By age 60, about 60 percent of Americans have it." Dr. Barry Marshall and J. Robin Warren have said that 70 percent of people with stomach ulcers have this bug (although other estimates have been from 40 to 60 percent), that 95 percent of people with small intestinal ulcers are infected with this bug, and that perhaps *almost half the people with other gastrointestinal problems* may have this bug.

Are Your Children Infected?

By the age of ten, 60 to 70 percent of children in developing countries are infected with this organism. It used to be called *Campylobacter* in children. An Italian study in *The Lancet* medical journal discussed thirty-two children averaging twelve years old who had *nonspecific chronic abdominal* discomfort. *All* were positive for *H. pylori.* One month after treatment, thirty of these children (90 percent) were better. In another study, Dr. G. Corrado and his Italian research team found that *H. pylori* infection in children *is commonly associated with food allergy.* At the other end of the human spectrum, *H. pylori* is a common cause of loss of appetite and burning sensations in the elderly.

How does this bug survive in stomach acid? These are very creative bugs. They survive in the acid environment of the stomach by producing their own alkaline shields. This protects the bacteria but still allows them to cause local infection. *H. pylori* also appears to occur in the mouth, so avoid kissing and sharing food during active infection.

How Do You Know if You Have an H. Pylori Infection?

A blood test and a new breath test can detect antibodies and demonstrate infection. If you are found to be infected with *H. pylori,* go on a program and rerun the test in eight weeks. Once you have a normal (negative) test, meaning you have no more evidence of this bacterial infection, you should have the test once a year for the next several years. Relapse of this bacterial infection may be one of the causes of high relapse of ulcers and gastrointestinal upset in general.

If you have ulcers or gastritis, or have had them in the past, you should get tested for *H. pylori*. Any kind of *chronic stomach and intestinal* problem that does not respond to customary treatment should be tested for this organism. *H. pylori* is also *so* often associated with stomach cancer that antibiotics are recommended as an inexpensive first line attack for early stomach cancers. *H. pylori* is now being researched for its link to other problems such as heart, skin, and eye disease. Since it is contagious, if any members of your household have it, you should be tested.

What to Do if You Have the Ulcer Bug

Medical treatment uses antibiotics and bismuth salts (classically found in Pepto-Bismol but now available in health-food stores without food dyes and sugar). *Antibiotics used for these bugs are Biaxin, amoxicillin, tinidazole, and metronidazole.* After antibiotic treatment, use nutrients mentioned earlier in this chapter. Treating *H. pylori* prevents relapses of ulcers in many cases.

Why add all the nutrients after the antibiotics? The rate of recurrence of ulcers is high. After eradicating *H. pylori* infection and then using DGL, recurrence is 14 percent. This is close to results achieved with ongoing antibiotics (but is higher when people go off the antibiotics). Since licorice extract is less expensive and less toxic than antibiotics, it is a sensible conservative approach to prevent recurrences. Use it for two to six months along with the other mentioned nutrients.

Some scientists believe *H. pylori* is an innocent bystander rather than the true cause of peptic ulcers. So just using medications to get rid of the bug is not a complete strategy.

When I was in practice, I ran *H. pylori* tests on anyone suspected of having ulcers or who had chronic digestive problems. At that time, I suggested DGL, bismuth salts, probiotics, and antioxidants, and then retested the patients. Seven out of ten patients got rid of *H. pylori* with this treatment. If they did not stay on some kind of a preventive program, some relapsed. But with healthful maintenance, most of them fared well.

Ask Your Doctor about Bismuth Salts

Ask your doctor to consider *bismuth salts* along with antibiotics. These promote a protective layer in the stomach and halt the growth of *H. pylori* without reducing the amount of acid that your stomach makes. Some studies comparing the treatment of *H. pylori* with antibiotics versus bismuth salts demonstrate that bismuth salts appear to be more effective than antibiotics. One article in a Scandinavian medical journal showed that bismuth salts helped heal the damage to the lining of the intestinal tract better than did typical ulcer drugs like cimetidine.

The dosage used in these research studies was 120 mg of bismuth four times daily, 20 minutes before each meal and before bed, for six to eight weeks. Bismuth salts may make your stools a little black. Some people may have a little diarrhea, headache, or dizziness, which usually goes away in several days as the body acclimates. Bismuth should not be used if you are on tetracycline, have kidney or liver problems, or are pregnant. Antacids and milk should not be taken within 30 minutes of taking bismuth salts as they will reduce its effectiveness.

Why Antiulcer Drugs Fail

Antiulcer pharmaceuticals reduce the acid environment of your stomach, allowing temporary healing of the ulcer, but they also cause a number of negative side effects. They deprive your body of acid, which is necessary for digestion, for protection against unfriendly bugs, for good bone health, and for turning on the rest of your digestive enzymes. These drugs may block good prostaglandin production, which can cause more inflammation and cellular damage in your body. They can damage your gastrointestinal lining, which can block digestive enzymes. And many of the antiulcer medications (H2-receptor blockers) promote the growth of all kinds of viruses, bacteria, and fungi, such as *Candida albicans* (yeast), which normally would have been killed in the stomach, to survive and colonize in the intestinal tract. (Women seem more prone to this than men.)

Most important, there is a high rate of relapse with pharmaceuticals. One study in the *British Medical Journal* revealed an 80 percent relapse after one year, and a 100 percent relapse after two years. Another study in the same journal showed that people maintained on treatment had an almost 50 percent relapse rate after one year.

Also, a number of acid-suppressing drugs cause acute liver damage; cimetidine was found to be the one most associated with developing this problem, from a study of over 100,000 ulcer-drug users.

Healing Your Ulcer

- *Test for H. pylori.* If you have the bug, doctors usually treat with antibiotics for two weeks and then switch over to natural protocols for maintenance and prevention. And remember, tests are not foolproof. Some doctors choose to treat on the basis of symptoms in the face of negative test results.

- *Eliminate stressors and increase protective factors* (see chapter 1).
- *Avoid aspirin and NSAIDs* with active ulcers. If you have a history of ulcers and you need these medications, ask your doctor about taking DGL, zinc, and fish oil to protect against injury to your intestinal lining.

If you have chronic or recurring ulcers:

- Identify and avoid allergic foods (see chapter 17).
- Insufficient digestive enzymes may be aggravating your problem.

One-Month Healing Program for *Mild and Moderate* Ulcers

You are encouraged to:

Eat smaller, more frequent meals and try to rotate foods. Eat softer foods (blended foods, juices, soups, and applesauce). Spicy foods? This depends on how you react. Studies show that red chiles do not make ulcers worse.

Eat more fiber foods. Make sure your diet includes high-fiber foods as well as some *soluble* fiber foods—psyllium, legumes, and pectin (like applesauce and apples)—not just whole grain breads and pastas.

Eat more fresh vegetables, especially green vegetables like cabbage, Brussels sprouts, and broccoli. If you don't like to eat these, take supplements with green vegetable concentrates.

Take a buffer drink on rising and before going to bed. This is a high-fiber drink (2 teaspoons of a high-fiber source plus 1 tablespoon of aloe vera juice mixed in a large glass of water or diluted juice, followed by a second glass of plain water).

Drink healthy juices, with an emphasis on cabbage. (Fresh cabbage juice, 1 quart a day, in five divided doses for the first week. You can add apples or other fruits for better flavor. Or take 1 teaspoon of vegetable powder containing cabbage, five times a day stirred in water.

Drink room-temperature liquids—cold and hot liquids tend to slow down emptying of the stomach.

Avoid dairy products. Use milk substitutes, such as those made from rice, almond, and soy.

Avoid alcoholic beverages, especially fermented ones like beer and wine; caffeinated beverages, tea, too much salt, chocolate, fried foods, and animal fats. If it is too hard to avoid, at least cut back.

Try eliminating wheat, citrus, and foods containing peppermint. Eat less animal protein, such as red meat, for one month, as it stimulates acid production more than vegetable sources of protein (such as soy products, beans, seeds, nuts, and grains). Don't eat later in the evening. Eating dinner earlier, rather than closer to your bedtime, has been shown to keep stomach acid levels lower.

Avoid refined sugars. Read labels. Sugar is hidden in many foods, such as ketchup, sauces, processed meats, peanut butter, and breads.

Nutrients That Help Heal and Protect Against Ulcers

- *DGL: licorice extract.* Chew 2 380-mg tablets three to four times a day on an empty stomach or 20 minutes before meals. Chewable tablets are available at health-food stores. After improvement, reduce to 2 tablets twice a day. For maintenance, use 1 to 2 a day for several months.
- *Zinc picolinate.* 30 mg a day, balanced with 2 mg of copper a day. Numerous studies on animals and humans show zinc's role in ulcer formation and healing. Even patients with long histories of bleeding and unsuccessful surgery have improved dramatically with zinc supplementation. Zinc increases the defense system of the stomach.
- *Antioxidants.* Some studies suggest that vitamins A, C, and E may help protect against ulcers or inhibit some of the mechanisms by which ulcers "grow." Free radicals (oxidants) are implicated in ulcer formation. Studies show that low vitamin C levels in stomach tissue accompany stomach inflammation. Food additives, especially in meats (nitrites), may use up the C in stomach tissues.
- *Vitamin A.* 5,000 to 10,000 IU (higher dosages during more active stages). Do not take over 5,000 IU without a doctor's supervision.
- *Vitamin C.* Buffered, 500 to 2,000 mg a day in divided dosages.
- *Vitamin E.* 400 to 800 IU to protect stomach lining.
- *Vitamin B complex.* 50 mg of each. Studies in rats and humans link B_6 deficiency with ulcer formation.
- *Glutamine.* 1,500 to 3,000 mg in divided dosages on an empty stomach. Research showed glutamine assisted ulcer healing.
- *L. salivarius,* a probiotic that has been shown to inhibit *H. pylori* (in test tubes). Take 3 capsules three to four times a day.
- *Garlic.* The equivalent of two small cloves per meal has been shown to inhibit the growth of *H. pylori*.

Say Good-bye to the Old "Drink Milk and Cream" Diet

The accepted medical treatment used to recommend dairy products to help heal ulcers. This is no longer the case. As early as 1976, Dr.

Do not take pancreatic enzymes if you have an ulcer or an inflamed stomach.

Deglycyrrhizinated licorice (DGL) is an herbal extract of licorice that has been treated to remove the glycyrrhetinic acid, the hormone part of licorice. Removing this acid molecule makes DGL safe to use, even over long periods of time. DGL does not reduce gastric-acid secretions, but helps rebuild and regrow the protective mucous lining of the stomach. DGL has been shown in experiments to increase the life span of the cells that line all areas of the GI tract. DGL is also effective in certain people in preventing ulcer recurrence.

Unlike medications, licorice extract does not promote yeast growth. Studies have also shown that DGL plus aspirin inhibits gastric bleeding without diminishing the therapeutic effect of aspirin. In other words, you get less damage from the aspirin, but you still get the benefits.

In rare cases, loose bowels or headaches have occurred from DGL. Small amounts can conceivably interact with prednisone, hydrocortisone, or other cortisone-type drugs. It is not known if it is safe for pregnant mothers so *do not take during pregnancy.*

Andrew F. Ippolite and coworkers reported in the *Annals of Internal Medicine* that all forms of milk they tested were potent *stimulators* of stomach acid. Milk does buffer, but milk also promotes more acid production. Also, milk products are a common source of food allergens. This is a good example of how medical treatments run in trends just like fashion, and what is commonly accepted does not always turn out to be accurate.

Herbs for Ulcers

When there is *no H. pylori* infection, try one of the following:

- Mix equal parts of cayenne, turmeric, and goldenseal powders and put in capsules. Take two capsules two times between meals for two months. When the ulcer is healed, take one capsule once a day for two more months.
- Another herbal option: Take 15 drops of tea tree oil in juice twice a day. Follow with tea made from slippery elm bark (steep 1 teaspoon of herb in water for 20 minutes, then strain). Drink two to four times a day for six week.

Other Aids

- Take aloe vera juice (several teaspoons up to 1/3 cup in water or diluted juice between meals to coat and regenerate stomach lining).
- Flaxseed and evening primrose oils, 3 to 6 capsules a day (take extra vitamin E) and several hundred mg of L-arginine, an amino acid, taken 20 minutes before meals several times a day (but not during pregnancy).

One-Month Healing Program for *Severe* Ulcers

During the first two weeks, consume drinks and foods that are soft. Eat soothing foods like avocado, papaya, bananas, well-mashed yams and potatoes, well-cooked carrots, mashed zucchini, blended spinach leaves, and cooked turnips. If you don't want to go through this effort, buy organic baby foods. Soft foods give your intestines a rest.

Easy Homemade Veggie Soups and Soothing Foods

Steamed Veggies   Steam vegetables such as carrots, yams, onions, zucchini, etc., then blend with the water you steamed them in and a little butter. Add salt or soy sauce to taste. Eat as a soup.

Ulcer Smoothie   Put a banana, an apple without the skin, and one helping of The Ultimate Meal in a blender. Fill with soy or rice milk or diluted fruit juice. Blend and enjoy.

Ulcer Pudding   Put cooked brown rice in a blender with rice milk, add vanilla and/or cinnamon to taste. Blend and eat with a spoon.

Juices and Soup for Ulcers

The emphasis is on cabbage juice. Cabbage juice is high in vitamin U, a substance (unknown to many people) that has been suggested to prevent the development of peptic ulcers and helps to heal peptic ulcers that are already formed. Garnett Chency, M.D., of the Stanford University School of Medicine research laboratories, found cabbage juice cured 95 percent of peptic ulcers in a hundred patients within two weeks. Follow-up studies have been inconclusive.

Note: Do not heat or store the cabbage juice. Drink it right away as the helpful factors in cabbage juice are quickly damaged. If you use a Vitamix or blender you get the juice along with the fiber, but add extra water when blending.

Early Morning Juices for Ulcers

- Juice orange, apple, celery, and half a head of cabbage (green is best).
- Juice half a head of cabbage, apples, carrots, and ginger.

Midmorning, Afternoon, and Evening Juices

- Juice cabbage, cucumber, ginger, and celery.
- Juice half of a cabbage plus Granny Smith apples, some fresh mint or parsley leaves to taste.
- Juice half a cabbage, tomatoes, garlic, broccoli, and carrots to taste.

For those who don't like juices:

Cabbage Stir Fry   Sauté cabbage and diced onions in a little butter or olive oil. Add salt and pepper to taste. Add grated carrots, pineapple, and optional turkey, chicken, or tofu. Serve over rice or noodles, or roll up in thin whole-grain tortillas (spread with plum or hoisin sauce first).

Mind-Body Techniques

Reflex Points for Ulcers

Use your thumb to explore under the ball of the left foot. Find the sorest spot and work that area for a few minutes. Then hold it. Breathe into your upper abdomen and stomach, relaxing these areas. Also explore the big toes to work out any sore or nodular spots. (See foot reflexology charts on pages 216–218.)

Two Easy Home Exercises

1. *Lazy Ulcer Exercise.* Lie on your back on the floor with your legs up on the bed. Twist your arms to your right, keeping both shoulders on the floor as best

you can. Then twist your arms to your left. Begin a swinging motion back and forth across your body at the level of your upper chest. Breathe in to the left side, exhale to the right side. Keep this up for one or two minutes the first few times, then increase to five minutes. Be careful not to get dizzy. Go slowly. Sit quietly for the same length of time after the exercise.

2.   *Ulcer Cobra Pose.* Lie on the floor on your stomach with your hands by your armpits and your elbows up toward the ceiling. Slowly push your palms against the floor, and lift your head and shoulders forward and upward. Lift yourself up as high as you can, while keeping your stomach and waist on the floor. *Do not strain.* Push your palms against the floor and try to create the sensation that you are tractioning your abdomen in the direction you are facing, lengthening it out and away from your waist. This is a healthy stretch for the abdominal area and enhances circulation and healing of this area.

Meditation

Blue Light Breathing. Sit relaxed. Take three breaths. Hold both hands over the upper abdomen. Inhale blue cooling light into your lungs (visualize the air you are drawing into your lungs as colored blue and "feeling" cool). On the exhale, visualize this blue light as traveling into your stomach and intestines, coating them with healing. Do this exercise for about ten minutes. Then sit and enjoy the silence for several more minutes. Healing takes place in silence.

Affirmation

Lie down. Take three deep breaths to get relaxed. Then begin slow inhales and exhales, saying affirmations on each part of the breath.

Inhale and say (to yourself), *"I smile."*

Exhale and say, *"I relax my stomach."*

Mindful Living

There is nothing wrong with having emotions of anger, resentment, or blame. *It is holding on to these emotions that is harmful.* Be mindful of letting "negative" emotions move through your body and thereby preventing them from getting stuck in your belly. Experience your emotions, then let them go.

An excellent way to self-monitor your anger:

When you are in a car, if someone else cuts in front of you or causes a small inconvenience, what is your immediate reaction? Protected by our cars, we often let out our below-the-surface anger. If your first response is to swear, yell, and demonstrate anger, this is a good indication that you have some general anger housecleaning to do. This anger may be keeping heat in your stomach and maintaining your ulcer.

13   *Healing Gallbladder Disease*

You've heard the expression "You have a lot of gall." The term *gall* comes from the Latin, meaning *bile.* The gallbladder is the storage vessel for bile. It is a small, pear-shaped organ that hangs behind and between lobes of the liver. The liver secretes bile continuously, but bile enters the intestinal tract only when needed. As a reserve, the gallbladder concentrates about two cups of bile and holds it ready for action.

Why do the liver and gallbladder go to this trouble to produce and stockpile bile reserves? Because bile helps break down fats, an essential process for the digestion of fat-soluble vitamins (A, E, D, K, carotenoids) and essential fatty acids. To digest fats, bile contains bile salts. These break fats into tiny globules, resulting in an emulsion—very similar to the homogenization of milk. This emulsifying action prepares fats so that pancreatic enzymes can work on them to further the digestion. Bile contains bicarbonates (baking soda) that buffer stomach acid, and this enhances digestion in the intestines. Bile also carries waste products from the liver. Thus, bile is an essential tool of *detoxification.*

When you eat fatty foods, they pass through your stomach into the upper part of the small intestine. A hormone (cholecystokinin) signals your gallbladder to squeeze bile into your intestines. This tells your liver to produce more. As you can see, the liver and gallbladder work closely together.

Most people ignore their gallbladder. They assume that if something is wrong with it, they can simply get it surgically treated or removed. But this is not the whole story.

TWO FRIENDS WITH GALLBLADDER PROBLEMS

John and Mark were the best of friends. They worked hard, played hard, drank a lot of beer, and ate fries on most Friday nights. They were both in their forties, a little overweight but strong as bulls.

But then the oddest thing happened. Within several months, they both had gallbladder attacks and ended up at the same hospital getting sonograms. Their doctors shook their heads when they saw the stones on the X rays. Laser surgery was recommended to both men, but Mark's wife, Gina, was an avid health-food person. She had read that gallbladder problems were often allergy problems. Through dietary means she helped Mark find out which foods were most likely the guilty ones. She gave Mark digestive enzymes. They shared reflexology treatments at night. Soon Mark's indigestion stopped. He didn't have any more attacks, unless he "sinned" and ate his allergic foods, which turned out to be eggs and pork.

John didn't want to bother with the "allergy thing." It seemed like way too much work and too far out, so he had the surgical procedure. John thought it had to be easy, because so many people have had it, but it took him longer to heal than he thought it would and his digestion never completely recovered.

Two solutions to the same problem. One surgical, one lifestyle. Healing the cause of your problem is more work in the short run, but better for your health in the long run.

What Can Go Wrong with the Gallbladder?

Potential problems of the gallbladder are:

- The gallbladder can get inflamed (cholecystitis).
- The ducts of the gallbladder can swell, causing bile to reflux back into the gallbladder and putting the gallbladder into spasm.
- Gallstone formation can cause the blockage of a duct, impaction, and sometimes infection, although gallstones probably don't cause as many of the problems with gallbladders as was previously thought.
- Attacks (severe episodes) make the gallbladder spasm just like a muscle, causing pain.
- Repeated attacks leave the gallbladder scarred, thick-walled (fibrotic), and unable to function normally.
- Stomach acid and fat stimulate the hormones that make the gallbladder squeeze. If you are low in stomach acid, you may not get adequate stimulus to the gallbladder, which can then start to *back up*.

The Earliest Signs of Gallbladder Problems

In early stages, gallbladder problems are usually free of symptoms. Even people with large gallstones may be symptom-free. By the time signals appear, the gallbladder disorder has usually been going on for a long time. In other words, if you have symptoms of gallbladder problems, you most likely have not been adequately digesting fats or fat-soluble vitamins for some time.

If you ignore recurrent gallbladder attacks, the gallbladder gets scarred, shrunken, and often adheres to the surrounding tissues, causing more chronic pain and problems.

Problems in the gallbladder usually show up first as *stomach problems*.

Symptoms Suggesting *Chronic* (Long-Term) Gallbladder Problems

- Indigestion (colicky upper-abdominal feelings), especially after eating fried, fatty, oily, and rich foods.
- Chronic gas.
- Chronic belching.
- Chronic abdominal distention and bloating.
- Fatigue. Gallbladder problems increase the toxic load that can gain entry into your body, promoting liver stress and free radical formation, which can cause sluggishness.
- Irritability and bad temper.
- Tendency to headaches and getting sick easily; gallbladder-induced toxic load can suppress the immune system.
- Anxiety.
- Sometimes a person with gallbladder illness will have no symptoms.

Symptoms Suggesting *Acute* (Severe) Gallbladder Attack

- Pain in the upper right abdomen radiating to the shoulder blade on the right side and/or shoulder and neck.
- Nausea, vomiting, severe pain.
- Severe pain, especially after eating foods that spur the gallbladder to release bile. These are fried or fatty foods or fat-soluble vitamin supplements (vitamins A, E, D, and K).
- Recurrent attacks without a sign of gallstone formation on a sonogram highly suggest food allergies and/or digestive enzyme deficiencies as part of the problem.

Possible Causes of Gallbladder Disease

Some common lifestyle offenders that contribute to gallbladder problems are lack of regular physical exercise, being middle-aged and overweight, having had a number of children, having experienced a rapid loss of weight in a relatively short period of time, and skipping meals—especially breakfast. Women with fair skin also tend to be more at risk for gallbladder problems.

Other contributing factors are:

Overconsumption of refined sugars and carbohydrates. Diets high in refined sugar and carbohydrates inhibit the liver from making enough bile while saturating the bile with more cholesterol.

Overconsumption of fatty, fried foods and foods rich in animal fats. Constant demand on the liver and gallbladder to produce and secrete bile overtax these organs.

Underconsumption of foods that contain vitamins E, B and C. Animal and human studies suggest that inadequate levels of vitamin E may set the scene for gallstone production and, if adequate vitamin E is available, stones don't form as readily. B vitamins may assist the gallbladder in releasing bile. Foods high in vitamins E and B are whole grains, raw seeds, beans, and fresh vegetables.

Low levels of magnesium and folic acid, found in green vegetables, and inadequate fiber.

Birth control pills, if used for five years or more. Hormone supplementation increases the risk of many fat-associated problems, one of them being gallbladder problems. Birth control pills increase stone formation by increasing cholesterol secretion into the bile.

Hormone-Replacement Therapy (HRT) has been shown to cause gallbladder problems in a number of women.

Constipation or long intestinal transit time. Studies have clearly shown that constipation or slow intestinal transit time might increase the chance of gallstone formation from supersaturated bile.

Parasites cause infections that, in rare cases, can lead to a buildup of calcium-based gallstones. Bacterial overgrowth can cause malfunctioning, too.

Inadequate stomach acid. Gallbladder sufferers can have stomach problems caused by inadequate levels of hydrochloric acid. Symptoms of bloating, belching, indigestion, heartburn, and gas are often helped by stomach acid pills (see chapter 19). One study of fifty gallbladder patients showed that many had excessively low levels of stomach acid; when treated, they had a reduction in symptoms.

Food allergies are an unrecognized but common cause of gallbladder problems.

The work of Dr. Jonathan V. Wright and Dr. James C. Breneman has established the role of food allergies as causing gallbladder disease in some individuals. Dr. Breneman achieved an astonishing 100 percent cure rate of symptoms (not dissolving of stones) in his gallbladder patients by identifying and eliminating their allergic foods. Dr. Wright reports he has not had to refer any gallbladder patients for surgery if they identify and avoid or treat their food allergies.

The foods most likely to create allergic reactions are dairy (especially cow's-milk) products, eggs, wheat, coffee, pork, and onions, though any food(s) may be the culprit.

Bone Loss from Gallbladder Disease?

Undigested fat can combine with minerals (calcium and iron), preventing their absorption and enhancing the risk of bone loss (osteoporosis). Undigested fats melt and coat other food sitting in your intestines, such as carbohydrates and protein, which decreases digestion and absorption.

When you eat a food to which you are allergic, allergic complexes are formed in the body. They can travel throughout the system and affect various tissues adversely. These allergic complexes can attack the gallbladder and bile ducts. In response, swelling occurs, which halts or slows down the flow of bile out of the gallbladder. It is this "backing up" of bile that causes pain. This is one explanation of how some people who don't form stones can still suffer gallbladder pain.

Why doesn't everyone treat allergies instead of going for surgery? Because treatments follow the direction of medical opinion, based on the direction of prevalent medical school instruction. This is influenced greatly by whatever procedures are supported by supply and pharmaceutical companies. Over 500,000 gallbladders are removed each year. This is big business.

What to Do for Gallbladder Disease

Dietary Suggestions

Eliminate refined sugars, refined carbohydrates, and caffeinated beverages.

Drink plenty of water and healthy beverages between meals.

Identify and eliminate food allergies. Avoiding food allergies halts spasms, pain, and attacks, and prevents further stone formation. It does *not* dissolve stones that already exist.

Focus on whole, fresh foods with an emphasis on fruits, vegetables, and vegetarian sources of protein. Try rice and soy cheeses. The jalapeño-flavored ones are some of the tastiest. Many of these cheeses make great melted-cheese sandwiches.

Eat more high-fiber foods to normalize bowel transit time (see Fiber Cocktail on page 25).

Do not overeat.

Do not skip meals, especially breakfast. Missing meals or avoiding food for twelve hours or more has been shown to increase risk of stone formation.

Exercise and lose weight slowly and sensibly.

Go off synthetic hormones.

Monitor intestinal transit time (see chapter 1).

Digestive enzymes—assess if you need them, especially stomach acid (see chapter 19). Two-thirds of gallbladder-disease sufferers have been found to be low in stomach acid. Ask your doctor about the Heidelberg capsule test.

Supplements to Dissolve Stones

- *Vitamin C.* 1000 mg three times a day. Studies have shown a direct correlation between the amount of vitamin C in the liver and how well cholesterol stays in solution versus being made into bile salts.

- *Lecithin (phosphatidyl choline).* 500 mg daily for one to two months. (This has not been fully tested but is suggested as beneficial in clinical practice.)
- *Peppermint oil.* According to Dr. Jonathan Wright, 1 drop three times a day may help promote stone dissolution.
- *Vitamins E and A* help heal the mucous membranes of the gallbladder. Long-term use of these nutrients may help prevent new stone formation.
- *B vitamins.* Taking a multiple with 50 mg of each along with 100 mg of Vitamin B_6 and 3 capsules of *fish oil* twice a day has been shown to help keep cholesterol in solution, preventing stone formation.
- *Hydrochloric acid,* if you need it (see chapter 19).

Other Options

Lipotrophic supplements. These are formulas contain substances that normalize liver and gallbladder functioning. Many companies make variations. Products usually contain lecithin, (phosphatidyl choline), methionine, choline, and inositol. Other nutrients can be added, such as vitamins C and B, folate, as well as herbs such as black radish, beets, turmeric, artichoke leaves, greater celandine, and ox-bile. Products should have at least 700 to 1,000 mg of methionine and choline. Take 2 tablets twice a day.

L. acidophilus. 2 to 3 capsules two to four times a day.

Taurine. 500 to 1,000 mg two to three times a day. Taurine is a naturally occurring amino acid that is a normal component of bile. It appears to assist fat digestion by binding to particular bile acids, increasing their ability to break down fats. The body makes its own taurine from internal stores of the amino acid cysteine. Thus, taurine is considered a nonessential amino acid and is not often considered for supplementation by many doctors. However, certain health conditions, such as gallstones, have been associated with taurine deficiencies. Animal studies suggest taurine levels decrease with aging and that supplementing with taurine may prevent gallstone formation. So far, taurine supplementation for gallstones has not been studied in humans. Taurine seems to be well tolerated by most adults. No serious side effects have been seen at levels up to 3 grams a day.

Flaxseed oil, 3 to 5 grams a day (take more vitamin E when you add oil), for two months.

Potassium iodide—a prescription item—helps dissolve the cholesterol in stones.

Milk thistle and yellow dock. These herbs have been used for hundreds of years to treat liver and gallbladder problems. Take in capsules or standardized liquid extracts before meals, several times a day.

Diets for Gallbladder Conditions

In the United States, 20 percent of people over the age of sixty-five have gallstones and over 700,000 surgeries are performed a year. Allergy avoidance does not dissolve existing gallstones. Go on a six-month program. Consider a gallbladder flush (see directions below) once a month for three months.

Drink 8 to 10 glasses of water a day with 1 teaspoon of black cherry juice in each glass. Start and end each day with fresh carrot, beet, ginger, and lemon juice. Drink freely of catnip, dandelion, and fennel tea (use any or all of them). Drink black cherry juice diluted with water and a little lemon throughout the day.

Consume as much uncrushed foods (such as salads, fruits, and nuts) as possible.

For an *Acute Gallbladder Attack*

DAY 1   Eat no solid food. Drink just chamomile or catnip tea, filtered water, or sip apple-cider vinegar and honey in water. Chlorophyll can be added to the tea or water.

DAY 2   Add juices and grated root salads. Grated apple or zucchini may also be added.

Juices: Carrot, apple, beet root.

DAY 3   Add shredded vegetable salads, fruit salads, yogurt, (a nice mixture is yogurt plus fennel seeds and fresh lemon juice) and uncooked blended apples (homemade applesauce). You may also add ground seeds, nuts, and some well-cooked grain, such as millet, brown rice, or buckwheat. Try basmati brown rice.

Excellent Gallbladder Foods and Drinks

Root vegetables (red and yellow beets, celeriac root, Jerusalem artichoke, garlic, and potatoes), applesauce, pear and pear sauce, cherry juice, and broiled fish. Eat less animal fats.

Tasty Gallbladder Salad   Grate a little red beet, carrot, and Jerusalem artichoke and add to lettuce or watercress, along with finely diced celery. Add a dressing of olive oil, rice vinegar or balsamic vinegar, a little tamari, and granulated garlic. Optional: Grated ginger and/or mustard. Mix well.

Helpful herbs for teas are dandelion, ginger root, wild yam, parsley, and catnip. Or heat water and add 10 drops each of milk-thistle and yellow-dock extracts.

Gallbladder Cocktails   Juice one of each: apple, pear, beet, a 1-inch piece of ginger, and a peeled lemon. (Add dandelion leaves if you can harvest them from your yard or purchase them at your local health-food store.) You may substitute watercress for dandelion. If you have only some of these items, then use just those.

If you can't get fresh juice, take 2 tablespoons Biotta carrot juice, 2 tablespoons Biotta beet juice, and the juice of a fresh lemon, mixed with enough water to make a full 8-ounce glass.

If You Have No Gallbladder

If you have no gallbladder, then you have no place to store bile, which is needed to digest fats. The liver is still making bile, but the bile "piggy bank" is gone. Immediately after gallbladder surgery, take digestive enzymes with added bile for two to three months with fatty meals, and some extra vitamin B_{12}.

Gallbladder Flush

Gallbladder flushes are effective *folk methods* to flush out the liver and gallbladder in order to enhance detoxification and healing. There are many variations. Some use olive oil and lemon juice, grapefruit juice, or magnesium sulphate (Epsom salts). The following is one I have used on myself and recommended to many others. Make sure you use only organic fruits, herbs, and filtered water while doing the flushes and *only to flush with medical supervision.*

If you have active gallbladder disease you must have a sonogram first (ultrasound). If your stones are large, do NOT do a flush, as the stones can get caught in the ducts and require immediate surgery. If you have small stones, gravel, or attacks without any signs of stones, you can do flushes. You may get slightly nauseated and experience stomach upset, or you may experience no symptoms at all. If you fare well, you can do a flush once a month for three to four months and then once or twice a year for the next two years. I do a flush as preventative care every few years.

Four-Day Gallbladder Flush

Morning flush: Four mornings in a row on rising, make a glass of fresh grapefruit juice. Add the juice of one lemon and 2 tablespoons of olive oil. Drink, then lie on your right side with your knees up for twenty minutes.

Eat at least four to five organic apples a day between meals. If you want to get a better overall cleansing, you can eat a clean diet of steamed or raw veggies and whole grains, and only olive oil, seasoned with tamari, Paul Bragg's Amino Acids, or Dr. Jensen's seasonings and garlic. But you do not have to choose to eat so *cleanly.*

Take 1 gram of vitamin C four times a day.

Evening flush: Start at 7:00 P.M. on the fourth night. Mix 1 pint of pure olive oil with the juice of 10 lemons. Take 1/4 of this drink every 15 minutes until it's gone. If you have nausea or vomiting, then sip a little cold pineapple juice (with some ice cubes in it).

You should be able to finish and get to bed around 10:00 P.M. You may wake up in the middle of the night needing to defecate, or at least feel like you need to, but this does not mean that anything is wrong. Repeat evening flush on rising.

What Comes Out? The flush can stimulate bowel movements, which will probably contain small, greenish, irregular pearl-shaped "stones." These small compounds vary in size from grape seeds to cherries. They are probably not gallstones from inside your gallbladder as much as congealed gravel that has been trapped. Clinically, their release is often associated with improvement in digestive and gallbladder symptoms, as well as enhanced energy.

What to Do After the Flush

You can choose to extend the benefit of the flush by adding a few more components for one more month.

Add daily: Milk thistle, garlic, vitamin C, and one serving of some green powder or chlorophyll source once or twice a day.

Diet: Once a day, have a few shredded beets and/or radishes (daikon, red radish, burdock root, or whatever you can get) with a little fresh lemon squeezed on top. Try to eat dark bitter greens like kale or chard at least three times a week. Eat at least two organic apples a day.

Excellent Post-Flush Juice   Juice a carrot, an apple, half a beet with some beet greens, a slice of ginger, and half a lemon. If you don't have beets, add 1 tablespoon Biotta beet juice. If you don't have a juicer, blend all these ingredients in a blender with organic apple juice and water.

Cleansing Enemas (Herbal or Coffee)

You may think that enemas sound like excessive or "antiquated" measures. However, they are useful tools of detoxification. You may choose to use other tools, such as herbs and exercise, which some consider to be more sophisticated methods. However, enemas are neglected tools of healing.

Coffee enemas were recommended in the *Merck Manual* until the 1950s. Peer review of medical literature about enemas and colonics is extensive. Enemas have been prescribed by physicians for decades. Studies performed with rats offer support that two substances in coffee enemas stimulate the release of bile and aid the liver in its detoxifying action.

Enemas for Gallbladder and Liver

Use only filtered water. Brew organic caffeinated coffee. Instead of coffee you may steep tea using any combination of the following herbs or any single herb: goldenseal, chaparral, dandelion root, catnip, or milk thistle. Put 3 cups of tea or coffee in an enema bag (purchased at any local drug store) and then fill the rest of the bag with water and stir.

Lubricate the enema tip with olive oil. Make sure your hands are clean when touching the tip. Lie on your right side and slowly insert the tip. Let half the fluid flow in slowly. Retain. Lie on your back. Massage the abdomen from left to right. Try to retain the enema for at least ten minutes. Release in toilet. Repeat with the second half of the fluid.

If you have chronic gallbladder problems, do an enema two to three times a week for one to two weeks, then once a week for two more weeks. You will not develop a dependency on them if you are also improving your diet, exercising, taking supplements, and making positive changes in your life. If you are doing only enemas, then you are not helping yourself and may develop an unhealthy dependency.

Mind-Body Techniques

Gallbladder Exercises

1. *Rock-a-Bladder.* Stand up. Make fists of your hands. Stick fists gently under your ribs on both sides. Maintain pressure and twist from side to side. This massages the liver and gallbladder. Do ten times or whatever is comfortable.
2. *Twist-a-Bladder.* Sit cross-legged. Put the thumb of your left hand under your right rib cage. Squeeze your ribs around your side with the rest of your fingers. Twist to your right, then rock back and forth, squeezing and massaging your right side. While you are doing this, inhale deeply. As you exhale, hum out loud and send this sound to the area under your hand (your liver and gallbladder). The sound should be a loud HUM that resonates throughout your body and into your rib cage. Repeat ten times or whatever is comfortable.

Reflex Points for Gallbladder

Rub, search, and find the tender and gritty points under the ball and big toe of the right foot, the liver point on the right foot, and the outer-middle area of both feet. Work these out until they feel less tender. Grittiness takes weeks or months to improve. Work on both feet, but concentrate more on the right one. (See foot reflexology charts at end of chapter 20).

Affirmations

Sit relaxed and quiet. Bring your mind's eye to your gallbladder, to your right side beneath your ribs. Be aware of how this area feels.

Take three deep breaths.

Inhale and say, *"Relax."*

Exhale and say, *"My gallbladder and liver."*

Inhale and say, *"Heal."*

Exhale and say, *"My gallbladder and liver."*

Inhale and exhale, repeating affirmations for as long as comfortable. Optional: visualize pink healing light filling and healing the gallbladder and liver area.

When you are finished, once again draw your awareness to your right side and your gallbladder. How does this area feel now?

Ancient Chinese Technique for the Gallbladder and Liver

Stand still but relaxed. Close your eyes. With your fingertips, pretend (visualize) you are pulling your gallbladder and liver out of your body and holding these organs several inches in front of you. Try to maintain this image until you feel a hollowness in your body, as if you had actually pulled these organs outside of you. Visualize these organs as green and healthy. Do this for five to ten minutes each morning for a month.

Face Acupoint for Acute Gallbladder Attack

Gently press above the middle of the right eyebrow for several minutes. Repeat several times a day for one month.

14 *Irritable Bowel Syndrome and Other Causes of Intestinal Pain*

- Irritable Bowel Syndrome
- Recurrent Abdominal Pain in Kids
- Sugar Intolerances
- Gut Pain from Nonsteroidal Anti-inflammatory Drugs
- Celiac Disease
- *Turista*
- Flu
- Caffeine Sensitivity
- Colicky Baby
- Leaky Gut

If you have chronic intestinal pain, discomfort, or digestive problems, ask your doctor to consider *H. pylori* infection, celiac disease, sugar intolerances, food allergies, parasites, candida-related complex, or any relevant problems mentioned below. Also, always consider your stress levels. Stress can create numerous intestinal symptoms.

Irritable Bowel Syndrome (IBS)

Unlike inflammatory bowel diseases (IBD), which are conditions of chronic inflammation in the intestinal tract, some of which are serious debilitating diseases (see chapter 11), irritable bowel *syndrome* (IBS) is one of the most common health problems that brings people into the doctor's office. In fact, half of all gastrointestinal complaints made to doctors are due to IBS.

The term "colitis" should really be applied only to inflammatory disease of the colon, whereas "spastic" or "mucous" colitis is more properly described as "irritable bowel," a condition in which there are no tissue changes such as inflammation or ulceration, yet the patient suffers with various symptoms. The most common causes are caffeine sensitivity, stress, milk allergy, and lack of fiber.

Common symptoms are various types of abdominal pain—from disagreeable vague pains to outright sharp ones, alternating constipation and diarrhea, erratic toothpaste-thin stools, gas, bloating, nausea, as well as seeing mucus in the stools. Other symptoms can be headaches, fatigue, anxiety, depression, and difficulty with mental focus. This condition is called a functional problem, meaning the gastrointestinal tract is irritable but for no known medical cause. Women are more frequently affected than men. This may turn out to be partly due to the fact that estrogen receptors (the signaling system for hormones) line the intestinal tract and hormonal fluxes in women may affect receptor-intestinal interactions and fluid fluxes within the gut.

Even though natural remedies offer a high degree of success, you need to see a doctor to rule out serious illness, especially if you have rectal bleeding, black stools, or mucus in the stools.

Types of Irritable Bowel Syndrome (IBS)

Spastic colon IBS. Symptoms are commonly caused by eating. Stools are inconsistent, passed a little throughout the day, and vary in size and consistency with alternating constipation and loose stools. The loose stools often occur in the evening. There can be sensations of incomplete evacuation, and mucus is often seen in the stool. A bizarre but severe rectal pain may accompany these symptoms (it feels like a hollow painful spasm up the rectum and there is sometimes difficulty sitting down), as well as headache, backache, colicky pain, or a long, dull ache which may be relieved by bowel movement.

Painless Diarrhea IBS. An urgent need to defecate, usually after rising and/or after meals, may not come with the pains mentioned above. The diarrhea with this kind of IBS does not usually occur at night.

Healing Your Irritable Bowel Syndrome

Avoid eating raw fruits and vegetables for the first week. Avoid sugar, refined carbohydrates, cow's-milk products, and caffeine for several weeks.

Nutrients for Irritable Bowel Syndrome

(one month program)
- *Enteric-coated peppermint.* 2 capsules three times daily, 15 to 30 minutes before meals (peppermint oil relaxes intestinal smooth muscle). Five scientific studies found peppermint oil to reduce the symptoms of IBS.
- *Fiber cocktail.* Once or twice a day (See chapter 2, page 25)

- *Glutamine.* 500 mg three times a day.
- *Magnesium.* Take 100 mg every several hours. Liquid Ca/Mg is excellent for this purpose. If your stools get loose, cut down on the dosage.
- *Probiotics,* like mixtures of *acidophilus.* Several capsules two to four times a day. Studies suggest that adverse fermentation in the gut may contribute to IBS and probiotics should help this.

Also Consider

Natural antispasmodics. See appendix B.

If you can't get any of the products listed, chew 5 papaya tablets every hour or take 100 mg of bromelain between meals two to four times a day for two days, or try several 50-mg capsules of valerian root extract two to three times a day.

After an attack, take licorice (DGL)—2 tablets chewed 20 minutes before meals) for one week.

If you continue to have problems, consider a bowel detoxification and rebuilding program (see chapter 20). Chronic IBS that does not respond to recommended treatment may indicate a parasite or fungal component (see chapter 15).

Identify food allergies or intolerances and eliminate these from your diet, especially if your IBS exhibits diarrhea. In one study of 40 patients with diarrheal IBS, those who complied with an elimination diet for two weeks (only 16 patients could comply) had a 72 percent improvement (see chapter 18). Some IBS has been shown to be due to allergies to brewers' and bakers' yeasts.

Soothing Juice   Juice celery, cucumber, parsley, and red apples. Dilute with water.

Soothing Soup   Cut up 3 potatoes and boil in water. Purée in a blender with a little butter and salt. Optional: Sauté celery and/or onions in a pan and blend with the potatoes.

Soothing Smoothie   Cut up banana and blend with organic soy milk or Rice Dream ice cream and a little water.

Recurrent Abdominal Pain in Children

One out of ten school-age children have recurrent abdominal pain. If intestinal disease has been ruled out by a doctor, many kids respond within one to three weeks to increased high-fiber foods in the diet (see chapter 2 for recipe hints). Kids who do not respond to fiber have been shown to become pain-free with *Lactobacillus plantarum*, taking 2 capsules two to four times a day for several weeks and then 1 capsule twice a day. Sauerkraut has plenty of *L. plantarum*—your child may be open to eating grilled cheese-sauerkraut sandwiches (but probably not).

Make sure your child gets tested to rule out *H. pylori* infection.

Intestinal Pain from Sugar Intolerances

Various types of sugars can cause problems in sensitive individuals, from intestinal disturbances like bloating and diarrhea to allergic reactions like swelling and rashes. Since these folks are intolerant to various sugars in their diet, these problems are referred to as *intolerances*.

Lactose Intolerance

The most common sugar intolerance is to the sugar found in dairy products called lactose. Lactose is a complex molecule that makes up a third of the calories in milk. Lactose is split, or digested, by an enzyme called *lactase,* which is manufactured in the intestinal lining. Inherited deficiencies, aging, or various traumas like parasites can decrease amounts of this enzyme. Lactase deficiency occurs between the ages of ten and twenty in 75 percent of peoples whose ethnic origin is other than northwest European. It affects 90 percent of Asians, 75 percent of American blacks and Indians, and many Jewish people.

Lactose intolerance is a common, undiagnosed form of intestinal trouble. If you consume dairy products but are not digesting them, this continued irritation can cause maldigestion, nutrient deficiencies, and food allergies. Symptoms of lactase deficiency can mimic some allergic symptoms. You may experience gas, bloating, diarrhea, and indigestion right after consuming milk products. Some people who think they are allergic to milk may actually be milk *intolerant,* owing to an absence of lactase. They may be avoiding milk products when they don't need to.

How to Identify and Treat a Milk Intolerance

Take some lactase tablets with milk products and see if that reduces your symptoms. If your symptoms greatly improve, this suggests you have lactose intolerance. Once you identify a milk intolerance, treatment is easy: Avoid milk products or take them with lactase enzymes. If you avoid milk products, take calcium tablets.

Many foods contain hidden dairy products. Watch out for foods that may have added milk products, such as breads, pasta, bagels, crackers, salad dressings, puddings, and sauces.

There are several tasty cow's-milk substitutes: Try rice, potato, oat, soy, nut, or seed milk.

Apple Juice and Pear Nectar

These juices have sugars that are difficult to absorb, especially for sensitive children, and are a frequent cause of childhood diarrhea. Eliminate these juices and substitute diluted grape juice, pineapple, orange, etc. Give various strains of Lactobacilli and/or yogurt for one to two weeks after the diarrhea to rebuild friendly flora. Intestinal gas, discomfort, and diarrhea can also come from fructose (added to many fruit drinks) in some sensitive folks.

Other Sugar Culprits

Mannitol artificial sweeteners in gums, candies, and foods can cause problems in sensitive individuals. Some of the new *healthy* sweetners can cause intestinal or allergic reactions. One syndrome is even called "chewing-gum intolerance"; it's caused by chewing large amounts of artificially sweetened gum. Symptoms like diarrhea and bloating can occur within an hour and last for 12 to 24 hours.

THE CHEWING GUM MYSTERY: SORBITOL IMBALANCE

A flight attendant, thirty-two years old, had doctors in a London hospital stymied. She suffered with severe chronic severe diarrhea and intestinal pain even though all her tests (blood, urine, and liver) were normal. The clue to her cure: She happened to tell the doctors that she chewed up to sixty sticks of gum a day. Each stick of the sugarless gum contained 1.25 grams of sorbitol. This meant she was getting up to 75 grams of this sugar substitute daily. As soon as she stopped her gum-chewing habit, the diarrhea and abdominal pain went away. This was reported in *The Lancet* medical journal.

This is a good reminder to look first at how we are living and eating for the answers to our health problems, especially intestinal pain, before getting expensive and exotic tests.

Gut Pain from Aspirin and Nonsteroidal Anti-inflammatory Drugs (NSAIDs)

These drugs can irritate the lining of the gastrointestinal tract and cause bleeding. Bleeding may be present even if you don't see black stools; you have to have more than a thimbleful of blood to be able to see black stools easily. NSAIDs can also affect normal sleep patterns by suppressing the sleep hormone melatonin.

While you are taking these medications, try healing nutrients to protect your intestinal lining:

Chew 1 to 2 DGL tablets 15 to 20 minutes before all three meals.

Take 3 fish oil capsules twice a day, and use chili powder in your food. A study of 18 people in Singapore showed that those who took 20 grams of chili powder in water before taking 600 mg of aspirin one-half hour later had much less stomach injury.

Chest and Abdominal Pain from Spastic Esophageal Problems

Arginine, 1 gram two to four times a day for a month, has been shown to decrease the frequency and intensity of chest pain attacks associated with spastic esophageal disorders without the adverse side effects seen with drugs for this problem. Don't take this amino acid if you are pregnant.

Celiac Disease

A wide variety of intestinal complaints—such as diarrhea, intestinal discomfort and pain, and bloating—may occur because of a genetic inability to digest *gluten*, which is found in wheat, oats, barley, and rye. This problem is called *celiac disease (CD)* and often goes undetected. Studies suggest its incidence is higher than expected. *This is important because untreated CD is associated with a doubling of mortality, largely due to an increase of cancer of the small intestine, which is preventable by adhering to a strict gluten-free diet.*

CD can occur in infants once they start to be fed foods with gluten, or it may occur at any age in adults. In women it often shows up from ten to fifteen years of age, with the first sign being anemia (blood loss can be caused by gluten damaging the lining of the intestinal tract). Other symptoms are weight loss, bone pain, numbness, water retention, and skin disorders. More commonly, children exhibit iron deficiency anemia and adults folate deficiency anemia.

If you suspect CD, ask your doctor about a new easy-to-perform antibody test called the *ELISA test for IgA anti-tTg*. However, you can try going off all gluten products for one month, then add these back in large amounts and see what happens. A return of your symptoms suggests you have CD. Substitute gluten grains with corn, quinoa, brown rice, spelt, and amaranth. Sometimes millet and buckwheat will not cause problems.

Silent celiac disease. In the majority of studies testing populations for celiac disease, it has often been found that one-third of the people tested who have the disease don't know they have it. If someone in your family has celiac disease, you have a higher risk of having it even without symptoms, and it is worth getting an antibody test to get this checked.

Turista (Montezuma's Revenge)

This temporary disturbance of your digestive tract is usually caused by exposure to "bugs"—bacteria or viruses your body is not accustomed to. Symptoms can be diarrhea, vomiting, fever, chills, abdominal pain, gas, and distention, all of which vary in severity and may last from one to three days or even weeks.

Treating Turista

- Don't eat for the first day.
- Take 2 citrus seed-extract capsules (250 mg) three times a day with diluted juice, or 1 oregano leaf and oil capsule three times a day with meals (whichever you can get). Do this for three to six days.
- Take 2 to 3 capsules of probiotics several times a day for one week, away from the citrus seed-extract or oregano oil. Eat generous amounts of cultured products like yogurt.

To Prevent Turista. Put 5 to 10 drops of liquid grapefruit-seed extract into any questionable water that you drink, consume probiotics generously, eat yogurt several times a day, and take 1 multiple digestive enzyme with meals.

Good probiotics to take while traveling:

- *L. sporogenes* does not need to be refrigerated and can be used for prevention and/or treatment.
- *Saccharomyces boulardii,* a nonpathogenic yeast originally isolated from the surface of lichee nuts, is a common European remedy for treating and preventing *turista.*
- Mixtures of various lactobacilli, if you have access to refrigeration.

If you get a rash, your problem lasts longer than three days or reoccurs, or if you get a high fever, see a physician. You may have caught a specific bug that requires a specific treatment.

Constipation While Traveling

While traveling, take probiotics several times a day or consume yogurt once a day. Take several fiber capsules with a large glass of water before bed. If this doesn't help, try taking 1 to 2 multiple digestive enzyme plus a multiple vitamin/mineral with each meal. Don't forget to drink adequate fluids.

Yeast Allergies and Unidentified Allergies Causing Tummy Upset

Never forget that undiagnosed food allergies can cause many nonspecific gastrointestinal problems. Allergic reactions to bakers' and brewers' yeasts are good examples. Elevated antibodies to yeast have been identified in numerous patients with *indeterminate colitis, irritable bowel syndrome, Crohn's disease, and ulcerative colitis.*

The 24-Hour Intestinal Flu

This is a temporary inflammation of the intestinal tract (gastroenteritis), sometimes called "stomach flu." It can be caused by a number of possibilities: food poisoning, specific viruses, emotional upset, too much alcohol in your system, and sensitivity to certain foods, drugs, or chemicals.

Symptoms include: sudden abdominal pain, diarrhea, vomiting, fever, and chills, all of which can vary in degree and last from one to two days.

Treatments for Stomach Flu

Try several of the following for one to two days:
- *Stop eating* until symptoms calm down.
- Have a commercial *soothing herbal formula* on hand and take every hour as needed (see appendix B, page 223).
- Eat *yogurt* generously.
- *Curing pills* (inexpensive Chinese herbs) are excellent to keep on hand. Take a whole vial with hot tea.
- *Bromelain.* 1 500-mg capsule on an empty stomach, three to five times a day.
- *Herbal mixtures.* 1/4 teaspoon each turmeric powder, ginger root powder, and fennel powder, mixed with unprocessed honey.
- Chew 5 to 10 chewable *papaya enzymes* with a strong cup of peppermint tea or hot water.

Caffeine Sensitivity

Caffeine can cause abdominal upset and nervous stomach as well as irritable bowel syndrome. Some people are sensitive even to one cup a day and don't know it. And many of us overconsume caffeinated beverages throughout the day. Remember, colas and tea, even green tea, have a fair amount of caffeine.

Caffeine abuse often goes undiagnosed. Symptoms include *loose stools in the morning, a furry tongue, and a jittery stomach prone to colicky pain, gas, and symptoms of IBS and maldigestion.*

Try a caffeine test. Taper down over a week from all caffeinated food products (even chocolate!) and then abstain for a second week and see if your symptoms go away. (Caffeine withdrawal may cause headaches.) Or, don't drink coffee first thing in the morning on an empty stomach. Try drinking it later in the morning or afternoon.

Morning Coffee Alternatives

One of my favorites is Caffix. Mix one heaping teaspoon of Caffix with hot water. Add milk or Vita Soy's Organic Vanilla Delight.

Other coffee substitute ideas: Raja antioxidant tea, hickory coffee, or Teecino Mediterranean Herbal Expresso that gets brewed right in your coffeepot like coffee.

Menstrual-Associated Gastrointestinal Problems

Hormone receptors for estrogen line the intestinal tract. Signaling of these receptors may affect fluid fluxes and this may be why some women get constipated or have loose stools, on a cyclic basis, before the onset of their menstruation. It may be helpful to take 50 mg of vitamin B_6 and 50 mg of magnesium, from midcycle to the onset of the period, along with fiber cocktails (see chapter 2) one to two times a day to normalize intestinal transit time during the premenstrum.

Colicky Baby

The most common causes of colic in babies are:

- Baby is breast-fed and is reacting to something in mom's diet. The most common culprits are cabbage, Brussels sprouts, cauliflower, broccoli, onions, chocolate, or cow's milk. Cut out whichever applies to you, or all of them, and see if baby's colic goes away.
- Allergies to something in the baby's formula (soy, oils, dairy, etc.).
- Vitamin B deficiency. You can give low-dose liquid B, which you can purchase at health-food stores, in baby's formula. Check with your doctor.
- The baby may need chiropractic or osteopathic care to correct problems in the neck, spine, or skull resulting from the birthing process. I knew one couple who had a baby with colic. They all suffered for a year; nothing

they tried worked. Though this may seem incredible, after one spinal adjustment the baby's colic immediately ended.
- There are a number of commercial remedies that work about half the time.

Leaky Gut Syndrome

This is an intestinal problem in which the normal barrier function of the intestinal lining has gone haywire. The intestines become too permeable, referred to as "leaky." Remember, your intestinal tract contains the outside of the world in the middle of you. If your intestinal lining is too porous, undigested large protein molecules and toxic substances gain entry inside the body and may burden the liver, immune system, and other tissues. These substances can cause many health problems, such as digestive problems, allergies, or even cognitive problems, such as autism in children.

Leaky gut can be caused by a disrupted balance of friendly and unfriendly bacteria; intestinal problems such as infectious agents, parasites, viruses, and bacterium; and other factors, such as the regular use of aspirin or anti-inflammatory drugs. Other causes may be food allergies or the inability to digest gluten in grains like wheat.

Have your doctor order an intestinal permeability test. (See appendix B.)

Helpful Nutrients for Leaky Gut (One-Month Program)

- *Lactobacilli mixture.* 2 to 4 capsules three times a day.
- *Glutamine.* 500 mg two or three times a day.
- *Vitamin A.* 5,000 IU once day.
- *Vitamin C.* 1,000 mg twice a day.
- *Vitamin B complex.* Once a day.
- *N-acetyl cysteine.* 30 mg once a day.
- *Fish oils.* 3 capsules twice a day.
- *Zinc.* 20 mg once a day.
- Consume foods rich in *flavonoids, fiber, carotenoids,* and *lycopenes.* (See chapter 1 about protector and stressor foods.)

Food Poisoning

Symptoms include severe stomachaches, vomiting, fever, constipation, and/or diarrhea within twenty-four hours of eating. Take oregano leaf and oil extract (three times a day with meals), activated charcoal, and yogurt or *L. acidophilus* several times a day, and stop eating solid food until everything is calm again.

See a doctor *immediately* to rule out salmonella or *e. coli* 157 infection if your fever goes over 101°F, if bloody diarrhea is present, or if your other symptoms don't go away in several days.

Chronic Abdominal Pain without Disease

Chronic abdominal "pinpoint" pain, meaning you can exactly point to the source, is difficult to diagnose. Consider hernias, "trigger points," referred pain, or pain from internal scar tissue. See a surgeon to rule out hernia, and for other possible causes see hands-on doctors, such as chiropractors or osteopaths. Sometimes acupuncturists can help. Also consider gynecologic problems and get a checkup by your gynecologist.

15 *Intestinal Invaders: Parasites*

You may think that parasitic infections only happen to people who travel to far-off places. But according to many specialists, parasitic infections are more common than was once believed, are not always easily detected, and should *always be considered when dealing with chronic intestinal diseases or chronic health problems.*

Renowned physician Dr. Sydney Baker stated at a conference that he didn't know how he managed to practice medicine before he knew how to diagnose and treat parasites. He said parasites can contribute to a wide array of health problems, especially chronic digestive complaints, along with many other health problems like arthritis, chronic fatigue, as well as problems with memory, anxiety, and depression.

NOT ALL STOOL TESTS ARE EQUAL

Helen had suffered with severe bowel disease for seven years. She had been on various medications, but nothing stopped her bloody diarrhea, which occurred numerous times a day. She also had severe fatigue, joint pains, and a haunting sensation of feeling constantly empty. Regular stool tests had never identified any harmful organisms.

Out of desperation, Helen came to see me, even though her own doctor did not approve of alternative medicine. I ordered a special purge test from a laboratory that specialized in parasites, explaining that parasites are not easy to find and that these unique tests give a better chance at detection. The laboratory diagnosed a parasite. Treatment of the parasite ended Helen's bowel disease within one month. The "empty" feeling and fatigue went away in two months. Her joint pain improved enough for her to start hiking again. *All* her symptoms had been caused by the parasitic infection.

Parasites? Not Me

A parasite is an organism that lives off another organism—you, the host. In acute infections, a person is usually alerted to an immediate problem by watery diarrhea, intestinal cramping, fever, and fatigue that occur within several days or weeks after being infected. But *parasitic infections may go undetected for months or years.*

Three Problems Associated with Chronic Parasitic Infections

1. *Vague gastrointestinal disturbances* include a variety of nonspecific chronic complaints, such as bloating, gas, altered bowel habits, and abdominal discomfort. *Parasites can mimic gastrointestinal problems, from irritable bowel syndrome to ulcerative colitis.* This does not mean that all ulcerative colitis is caused by parasites. It means that all cases of ulcerative colitis should be tested to see if a connection exists.

    Dr. Leo Galland, a renowned parasite specialist in New York City, reminds us that chronic amoebic dysentery can look just like ulcerative colitis and can evade diagnosis. Dr. Galland had one patient with a ten-year history of severe bleeding ulcerative colitis. This patient had annual exams that did not detect any parasite infection. After herbal treatment for parasites, the man's *alleged* ulcerative colitis disappeared. This proved that the man didn't have true ulcerative colitis; he had chronic amoebic dysentery that mimicked ulcerative colitis.

2. *Allergic/inflammation/immune problems.* Parasitic infection can create constant irritation and inflammation of the intestinal lining. This can promote all kinds of maldigestion, from inadequately digested food to sugar intolerances. Intestinal irritation and inflammation can then cause food allergies.

    In my practice, I found chronic *joint pain* to be one of the most common symptoms of undetected parasites. This is called "reactive arthritis" because the body is getting an immune reaction to the chronic parasite infection. This immune reaction commonly manifests in the joints and mimics arthritis.

HOW UNFRIENDLY BACTERIA CAUSED JOINT PROBLEMS

Steve was a construction worker. He carried, lifted, hammered, and used his body strenuously all day. One month he developed tendinitis in both his wrists and severe joint problems in his knees. He hurt so badly he had to go on workman's compensation. After four months of physiotherapy and proper safety instructions, Steve tried to return to work. But he still hurt and he became deeply concerned about being able to continue the only job he knew and loved.

Steve came to see me. After taking a detailed history, I discovered that one of Steve's children had been treated for *Giardia* (a prevalent parasite) the previous year. Although Steve didn't have any intestinal complaints, we ran a test. Steve was shocked to discover that he was infected. He was even more shocked to learn that intestinal bugs could be causing his joint pain.

Steve had a choice of going on medications to "kill" the parasites or an herbal nutritional program designed to rebalance his system. Steve decided to try the nutritional supplements first. After going on a natural program for five weeks, Steve's second test was normal and so were his wrists and knees. He was able to go back to work without any problems.

3. *Chronic fatigue* of unexplained cause. All chronic-fatigue patients should be tested for parasites. When parasites become embedded into the intestinal wall, they can give off toxins. As long as they are infecting the host, they keep giving off toxins and can do this for years. The immune system constantly has to defend against these toxins, which takes energy away from your immune system that should be available to fight off other invaders. This explains how persons with chronic undetected parasite infections can experience overall poor resistance, chronic fatigue, and low-quality health.

    Toxins given off by parasitic infections can also cause liver stress. This increases the production of free radicals (oxidants), which gain entry into the bile and pancreatic ducts. These refluxes cause pancreatic stress and enhance potential for malabsorption syndrome, which can cause food allergies (and intolerances) as well as promoting chronic fatigue symptoms. These problems may be accompanied by night sweats, unexplained bouts of fever or rashes, feelings of poor health, anxiety, chronic viral or flu symptoms, or depression for no apparent reason.

AIDS and Parasites

Scientific publications suggest the development of AIDS may be enhanced by intestinal parasites. The AIDS epidemic in San Francisco was preceded by parasite epidemics. High-risk people would probably benefit from a yearly antiparasite program. This may hold true for some other types of viral infections. See chapter 17.

Why Is It Difficult to Know if You Have Parasites?

Parasite infections are on the increase because of increased sources of contamination. Possible sources are widespread. People eat out in restaurants more frequently than ever before. More children attend day-care centers. Many food handlers are from other countries and carry different parasites. Pediatric and dental clinics have reported outbreaks. We consume more imported foods than in any other time in history. We also travel to other countries more frequently.

Other sources are improperly washed foods, raw fish and meat, pets, not washing hands after using public bathrooms or gardening, water contamination from swimming or drinking. It becomes obvious, reading this list, that sources for parasite infection are ubiquitous.

Parasites may go undetected for years because they may not produce serious symptoms, but rather low-grade ones that are not easily identified. Parasites go through different stages that may affect your body in varying ways and thus may be difficult to pinpoint. And parasite infection may go undetected because, until recently, doctors were not aware that parasites could mimic chronic illnesses such as digestive disease, arthritis, and immune disorders.

The Most Famous Critter

Giardia lamblia is such a common parasite that we will discuss it in detail. Two other prevalent parasites are *entamoeba histolytica* and *cryptosporidium*. Cryptosporidium is being seen more and more in city water because chlorine doesn't always kill it.

In most countries, 7 percent of the population is infected by *Giardia*. In some countries its presence is greater. It is the most common cause of parasite infection in the United States. Some studies show that 10 percent of food handlers in this country are infected.

No one really knows the exact way *Giardia* causes illness. Some of its side effects are due to the fact that it invades the upper intestines. Here it succeeds in damaging digestive enzymes (disaccharidase) that are formed in this area of the lining of the upper intestines. The most common enzyme that is damaged is lactase, necessary for digesting the simple sugar in milk. Thus, people with chronic *Giardia* infections often complain of gas, bloating, and discomfort after consuming dairy products.

Giardia can cause any of the other problems mentioned above. *Giardia* exists in two live phases: *trophozoite* (parasitic form) and *cysts* (inactive form in egg sacs). But *Giardia* does not have to be alive to cause problems; even dead *Giardia* bodies can give off toxins that damage enzymes.

Giardia infection can cause severe, chronic fatigue. Drs. Leo Galland and Herman Bueno found *Giardia* infection in 61 out of 218 patients who came to their clinic with the chief complaint of chronic fatigue. Curing the parasite resulted in getting rid of the fatigue. It even eliminated viral-like symptoms (flu feeling, abdominal discomfort, sweats, and muscle aches and pain) in 70 percent of the people.

Note: Being infected with several different parasites at the same time, or with *entamoeba histolytica* (which can be associated with serious complications) are urgent medical situations.

This suggests that Giardia may be a significant contributor to a number of chronic fatigue syndrome cases, as well as chronic viral-like illnesses.

All parasite infections, including *Giardia,* upset the intestinal ecology. This can create an "intestinal unwellness domino effect," causing a number of other problems. These include malabsorption, bacterial overgrowth, colonization of yeast (*Candida albicans*), nutrient deficiencies, and food sensitivities and allergies.

Giardia and other parasite infections can promote and may often accompany intestinal yeast infections. Both may need to be treated for the person to finally achieve wellness.

Testing for Parasites

Most physicians order a one-time random stool sample. This has a high degree of *inaccuracy.* Also, most labs don't test for a wide array of worms, bacteria, fungi, amoebae, etc. Use specialty parasite labs such as those mentioned in appendix B. These labs use purge tests, in which some kind of laxative helps loosen organisms embedded high up in the intestinal lining. No method of detection is infallible. Sometimes the best idea is to go on an antiparasite program and see if your symptoms decrease while your general health improves.

As Dr. Alan Gaby reminds us, listening to our bodies is often more helpful than only relying on expensive laboratory tests.

However, once you have had a positive test, detected by stool analysis, it is a good idea to repeat tests once a year for a while. Parasites are tenacious. They can recur and the symptoms of recurrences may vary and be confusing. Family members should be tested, too.

Parasite Treatment

According to experts like Dr. Leo Galland, herbal treatments for parasites, compared to medications, are often very effective, less toxic, and create fewer side effects. However, sometimes traditional medications are needed and it is a good idea to get doctor's supervision for whichever program you embark on.

For Parasites

- *Antiparasitic formulas* (numerous companies make excellent formulas) available at local health-food stores. The main ingredients often include Artemisia annua, berberine, and/or garlic.

- *Oregano oil.* 6 to 10 drops in a capsule with meals two times a day for six weeks. If in pill form, take three or four times a day with food.
- *Supportive herbs.*
- *Probiotics* like *L. acidophilus* are needed, as grapefruit-seed and olive extracts destroy good bacteria, too, so take 3 to 4 capsules three to four times a day during the treatment and reduce dosage to 3 capsules twice a day for one month after the treatment.

Artemisia Annua (Wormwood)

This herb comes originally from China and has been used in China and Europe for centuries to treat parasites. It contains a specific antiprotozoa substance called artemisin, which has been investigated at Walter Reed Army Hospital. Artemisia annua, in capsules and teas, is safe, but *avoid pure wormwood oil.* Artemisia annua is recommended by Dr. Christopher, a well-known herbalist, for treating pinworms and roundworms.

Take 1 or 2 capsules three times a day after meals for six weeks.

No herbs or nutrients should be used during pregnancy without a doctor's supervision.

Grapefruit-Seed Extract

This product is used widely in Europe in the treatment of intestinal parasites. Extract of citrus seed has broad-spectrum antimicrobial activity. According to Dr. Leo Galland, the way the ingredients are connected to each other, called a "bio-mass," gives the citrus extract its potency. It acts only inside the intestinal tract. It is considered safe and usually does not cause allergic reactions. However, some people have a really difficult time taking this. It should not be used without a doctor's supervision. It should be organic in origin and free of chemicals, and yogurt or probiotics need to be taken along with it and for one to two months afterward, as it kills friendly flora while it's killing the *bad guys.*

Dosage should be supervised by a medical doctor.

Other Herbs

Black walnut leaf extract helps halt and inhibit worm growth. Cloves, wormwood, and quassia herbs help in similar fashion.

Goldenseal. One of its active ingredients, berberine sulfate, is effective against parasites such as amoebae, and also soothes an irritated intestinal lining.

Garlic has antiparasitic and anti-inflammatory actions.

Jerusalem oak has been used to treat a variety of worms.

Oregano contains 30 active ingredients, 12 of which help combat parasites, fungi, bacteria, and viruses.

See appendix B for suggested products that contain King Solomon and Black Seed, also very helpful for these conditions.

Take Lactobacilli *or mixtures of probiotics when you take any of these herbs and generously consume cultured products like yogurt.* If you are dairy sensitive, eat soy yogurt, If you are soy sensitive, consume *Lactobacilli* products made without dairy or soy.

Possible Side Effects of Parasite Program

A possible side effect upon starting a program to eradicate parasites is a *Herxheimer reaction,* which produces an increase in your original symptoms, as well as fever or flu and/or viral symptoms the first few days after starting an antiparasite program.

When parasites are going through *die-off,* the dead organisms give off toxins that may create symptoms. These temporary symptoms, called Herxheimer reactions, *are actually good signs. It means the program is working.*

Herxheimer reactions usually last only three to four days and should not persist longer than five to seven days. If your symptoms persist, you may need other antiparasite products and/or a detoxification program. Tell your doctor.

After a Program for Parasites or Worms

Rebuilding Intestinal Flora and Lining

(For one month)
- *Vitamin A.* 5,000 IU once a day.
- *Glutamine.* 1 gram (1,000 mg) twice a day.
- *Folic acid.* 800 mg once a day.
- *B-vitamin complex.* Once a day.
- *Antioxidant formula.* 1 capsule twice a day.
- *Probiotics mixture* of *Lactobacilli* and other friendly bacteria. 2 to 3 capsules two to three times a day.

If You Do Not Get Well from Your Parasite Program

If your antiparasite program does not seem to be working, you may need antibiotics.

There may be overlapping problems of *candida,* food allergies, or specific nutrient deficiencies that are blocking healing (see chapters 16, 17, and 20). Assess need for enzymes (see chapter 19).

You may need liver support. Take milk thistle and/or yellow dock for one month.

Do a detoxification and rebuilding program (see chapter 20).

Consider working with a homeopathic doctor (a meticulous study on twenty patients at the King Health Center in Lowellville, Ohio, showed significant response with homeopathics in treating parasites). Read Dr. Leo Galland's book, *The Four Pillars of Healing.* It is a superb resource on parasites and healing.

Tasty Drinks to Enhance a Parasite Program

Parajuice #1   Juice carrots and apple and dilute water. Add half a dropperful of goldenseal tincture before drinking.

Parajuice #2   Juice tomato, garlic, onion, celery, and carrot. Add half a dropperful of black-walnut tincture.

Parajuice #3   Juice cabbage, carrot, and apples. Then blend with a handful of pumpkin seeds.

Parablend   Grind pumpkin seeds first and then blend with soy or rice milk.

Worms

Even though it's hard to fathom, people can have undetected worm infections in their gastrointestinal tract. These creatures can be smaller than one inch or greater than 25 feet in length and they can cause a wide variety of health problems. Regular stool testing is not a consistently reliable way of diagnosing worms. Most antiparasite treatment programs don't work for worms.

All family members should be treated simultaneously by your doctor if one person has worms. Worms often require a three-month program of medical treatment plus herbs. Ask your doctor.

According to herbal folklore, *pumpkin seeds* in large quantities help treat worms. Add 8 ounces of ground seed to fruit juice and blend. Children drink 8 ounces of this blend, and adults 16. Two hours later, take 2 tablespoons of castor oil and be close to a bathroom.

Sensible Ways to Avoid Parasitic Infections

Food

Wash fruits and vegetables thoroughly before cooking or consuming. Don't cut up other foods on unwashed cutting boards or with utensils that have been used on raw meat, chicken, or fish. Don't wipe kitchen counters with rags or sponges, use disposable paper towels. Wash your hands after handling raw meat, chicken, or fish, and avoid touching your mouth before washing hands.

Avoid eating raw beef and fish, especially if you have inadequate levels of stomach acid. Eat at restaurants that practice optimal hygiene. Don't drink local water while traveling in foreign countries. Take herbs, digestive enzymes, or friendly bacteria at least one week before and throughout foreign travel.

Pets

Wash your hands after touching pets. Don't kiss your pets on the nose or mouth. Don't let your pets sleep by your head or crawl around on your pillows or sheets. Wash bedding frequently if animals are allowed on the end of the bed.

Don't let your pets eat out of your dishes. Deworm your pets once a year even if they do not have signs of parasite infections.

Other Advice

If your child is in day care, consider getting several random stool samples if outbreaks of intestinal problems arise.

Wash your hands after going to the bathroom and after gardening.

Mind-Body Techniques

Reflex Points

On the feet, work all intestinal points, from the stomach to intestines to rectum. Find tender points, work these out for several minutes, then move on to the next point. Finish by rubbing the entire sole of each foot and the sides of the lower legs firmly with your knuckles. (See foot reflexology charts at the end of chapter 20.)

16 *The Candida-Related Complex*

Candida and its role in health and disease has become extremely controversial. However, from the work of respected physicians not afraid to find answers in unconventional places, and from years of personally treating numerous patients, I believe that the candida-related complex is a valid clinical entity. Dr. Leo Galland, a noted physician and educator who has treated hundreds of patients with candida-related problems, says there is impeccable evidence that this illness is real.

However, many people unjustifiably attribute their illness to yeast when this is not the case. For you who are suffering with this condition, there are dietary and nutritional supplement measures that help. This chapter is about shedding some light on *candida confusion*, and giving you "the rest of the story."

Dr. Truss Sleuths Out the Candidiasis Story

For the last several decades, Dr. Orion Truss has done a meticulous job investigating the disease entity of *Candida albicans* and reporting this to the medical community.

In the 1940s, Dr. Truss was practicing as Chief Resident in Internal Medicine at the Cornell University division of Bellevue Hospital in New York City, where they were testing many of the new antibiotics. He noted that many people given these antibiotics got severe diarrhea and yeast infections.

In 1955, Dr. Truss visited a man in the hospital who had been healthy all his life, up to the time he suddenly got ill for two weeks and was now close to death. No one could identify what was wrong. Many diagnoses were considered, even Hodgkin's disease. Dr. Truss studied the man's hospital chart. The only thing that Truss could find in the chart were two stool cultures positive for candidiasis. Dr. Truss gave the man a supersaturated solution of potassium iodide, which is one treatment for candida. In a short time, this man, who everyone thought would not make it, recovered. He then told Dr. Truss that he had cut his finger on the job, and had been given antibiotics for two weeks when his finger got infected. Two weeks later he had become ill.

In 1961, Dr. Truss was in private practice. His son had developed asthma, so he began working with desensitization methods for allergies. During this time a woman came to see him with chronic vaginitis. Dr. Truss gave her a desensitization vaccine for candida. She came back and reported to Dr. Truss that not only had her vaginal yeast infection gone away, but so had her chronic depression! Thus, Dr. Truss began to see a connection between infection with yeast and immune and psychological functioning.

Dr. Truss admits that we have more questions than answers. But we do know that candidiasis as a disease entity does exist, even though it is often not recognized by the allopathic medical community except in severely immune-compromised people.

What Is Candida?

Candida albicans is a yeast. A yeast is a single-celled fungus. The term *Candida albicans* comes from the Latin, meaning "glowing white," and it was so named because this yeast is white in color. There are 600 strains of candida, not all of which cause health problems. About 25 strains may pathologically affect humans.

Candida albicans is ubiquitous and covers everything that is living on this planet. It is a normal inhabitant of the earth, and the human body. Under healthy circumstances, candida is a normal fungal organism that cohabits along with us in a safe and delicate balance between host and organism. Under healthy circumstances, it does not cause health problems.

It is when this delicate balance is tipped that candida, which is normally *living in* people but not *invading* people, can grow out of control and create a wide array of mild to severe health disorders. When this happens, this is now a candida infection, which is referred to by a number of names—enteric candidiasis, systemic candidiasis, chronic candida albicans, the yeast syndrome, or candida-related complex (CRC).

Candidiasis

Yeast existing inside our bodies as a round-shaped, single-celled fungus does not cause health problems. When it changes shape, elongating into a hot-dog shape called a mycelia, these mycelia can embed or root into tissues and colonize (grow out of control). This is called a yeast infection or *candidiasis*.

Why does yeast grow out of control? When we are healthy, yeast are kept in check in the single-celled form. When we lose our robustness and balance in our intestinal and immune environments, yeast can turn into the more harmful myceliated forms and start to colonize.

What Is Candida-Related Complex (CRC)?

The traditional medical community recognizes candidiasis only as either a local infection of the skin or mucous membranes (such as vaginal yeast infections) or as systemic infections. Systemic yeast infections, in which yeast is carried by the blood throughout the body, are rare, occurring only in severely immune-compromised people suffering with conditions like cancer or AIDS.

Many natural doctors theorize that there is another type of infection that can occur with yeast. They suggests that when yeast grows out of control in the intestinal tract, it "burrows" into the lining. There the yeast creates continuous inflammation and can also give off toxins that are absorbed through the intestinal tract into the body. The inflammation and toxins put a strain on the immune system, taking its energy away from surveillance. The toxins, and allergic reactions to them, can cause a wide variation of symptoms throughout the body. And candida can create antigens. Antigens are foreign substances able to affect the immune system. Seventy-nine candida antigens have been identified.

This holistic theory presents candida as a systemic illness referred to as the *candida-related complex (CRC)*. But it is different from the medically recognized blood-borne infection. Rather, the yeast infection remains in the intestines. It is the effect of the absorbed antigens and/or toxins—and possible allergies to these toxins and/or the burden on the immune system from those toxins—that create the wide variety of symptoms that make up CRC.

Symptoms Associated with CRC

Symptoms of CRC can include such chronic digestive problems as bloating, diarrhea, chronic stomach inflammation, swelling of the tongue and lips, inflammation of the esophagus, heartburn, and rectal burning and itching.

Other symptoms include fatigue, brain fog and spaciness, headaches, muscle aches, chronic flulike feelings, sugar sensitivities and cravings, allergy symptoms (which can vary widely from headaches to chronic postnasal drip), and chemical and odor sensitivities.

CRC may be associated with specific problems:

- Chronic digestive problems.
- Chronic fungal infections of the skin and/or nails.

- Female disorders: chronic vaginal discharge, vaginitis, chronic inflammation of the urinary canal, premenstrual syndrome, endometriosis, painful breasts, and other hormone imbalances. The most common female sign is chronic yeast infections of the vagina.
- Male disorders: prostatitis (inflammation of the prostate) and benign prostatic hypertrophy (benign enlargement of the prostate). The most common male sign is chronic loss of libido not due to organic health problems.
- Central nervous system problems can include learning disabilities, agitation, and depression.
- Serious illnesses such as some cases of multiple sclerosis, schizophrenia, lupus, and psoriasis.
- CRC most commonly occurs when a person develops symptoms within a year of taking several rounds of antibiotics, as well as developing extreme sensitivity to sweets, sweet cravings, and fungal infections.

Clues to Figuring Out if You Have CRC

Candida-related complex is usually diagnosed on the basis of a questionnaire and, most important, by embarking on a treatment program and seeing if there is a positive response. A number of laboratories have various tests such as candida-antibody tests, but their interpretation is controversial.

Take this self-help questionnaire. If you answer Yes to six or seven questions, you have a fair chance of having CRC. If you answer Yes to eight or nine questions, your chances are moderate. If you answer Yes to ten or more questions, you have a significant chance.

CRC Questionnaire

1. Have you ever been on antibiotics for over three months at one time?
2. Have you taken antibiotics three or more times in one year?
3. Women: Do you suffer from chronic hormonal problems such as PMS, endometriosis, or cyclical painful breasts? Have you been on birth-control pills for over six months? Do you have chronic or recurrent vaginitis?
4. Men: Have you had an alarmingly lower sex drive than you used to without an appropriate reason?
5. Do you have chronic fatigue?
6. Do you smoke?
7. Do you take ulcer medication?
8. Do you take steroid hormones?
9. Do you drink more than three drinks a night on a regular basis?
10. Have you ever been an alcoholic?
11. Do you have diabetes, cancer, or AIDS?
12. Do you crave sweets and carbohydrates?
13. Do you often have night sweats or flulike feelings?
14. Is your short-term memory terrible?
15. Do you have chronic digestive problems?
16. Do you have excessive stress in your life on a regular basis?

17. Do you have bouts of severe depression that are not in harmony with who you are or what is happening in your life?
18. Do you have chronic anxiety?
19. Do you have frequent headaches?
20. Do you just feel "bad" much of the time and you don't know why?
21. Did much of your bad feelings start right after or the year after taking antibiotics?
22. Were you colicky as a child? Did you have chronic middle-ear infections? Did you have thrush?
23. Do you suffer from chronic asthma, eczema, or hives?

The Message of Candida

Candida, growing out of balance, has a message for us. This problem is alerting us that humans are *out of balance* with the environment. When the ecology of the world gets disrupted (by drugs, hormones, sugars, stress, chemicals, pollutants), the individual human ecology is disrupted. Then once-friendly inhabitants such as candida metamorphose into enemies that can create or contribute to disease.

Candida is a recent health problem that has been occurring since the 1940s and appears to be getting more prevalent because our natural balance with the environment has been disturbed.

Dr. William Crook, a noted practicing physician, eminent educator, and author of ten books, wrote *The Yeast Connection* based on this concept. He felt that the totality of our health is made up of a number of connecting factors, and when this network breaks down, candida may grow out of control.

In the twentieth century, a variety of exposures, stressors, and foods can disrupt this ancient friendly *treaty* between humans and candida. Among the disconnecting factors are:

Diets high in consumption of sugars, fruit juices, and refined carbohydrates. This creates an environment that can promote overgrowth of candida.

Repeated exposures to antibiotics: a ten-day to two-week round of antibiotic three to four times in one year; antibiotics for more than two months at one time; or tetracycline to treat acne for years. Antibiotics were initiating factors of this illness in 82 percent of 91 patients whom Dr. Galland studied for CRC. The

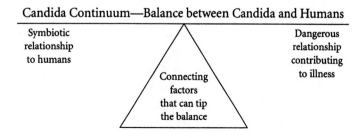

Candida Continuum—Balance between Candida and Humans

Symbiotic relationship to humans

Connecting factors that can tip the balance

Dangerous relationship contributing to illness

present-day excessive use of antibiotics and other immune-suppressive drugs is contributing to the tremendous increase of this condition. The standard American diet contains meats and dairy products that often contain antibiotics (animals are fed antibiotics on a regular basis to prevent disease).

Increased hormone exposures from: repeated pregnancies, hormonal imbalances, or birth-control pills (all of which can disrupt blood-sugar balance in the body), and chemicals in the environment that "mimic" hormones. Examples are dioxin in paper products and residues of DDT in foods found on grocery shelves. These types of hormonal exposures may promote an environment that encourages overgrowth of candida.

Premenopausal women with unopposed estrogen (elevated in ratio to progesterone) and women on hormone replacement therapy (HRT) are more at risk for CRC since estrogen increases the growth of *Candida albicans* and can shift the organism to a more virulent form.

Steroid hormone medications such as cortisone or corticosteroids (often prescribed for arthritic or dermatological problems).

Ongoing use of ulcer medications.

Exposure to tobacco.

Stress (chronic low-grade or isolated bouts) can depress the immune system.

Millions suffer with debilitating illnesses such as AIDS and cancer, which are often associated with increased growth of candida. Radiation and chemotherapy enhance yeast growth.

Infection with parasites can alter the intestinal environment and encourage the overgrowth of yeast. Every yeast-infected patient should be tested for parasites.

Do You Have Brain Fog?

Fuzzy thinking and poor concentration and memory are often associated with CRC. This is because yeast overgrowth can contribute to nutrient deficiencies, toxic reactions, and allergies, which can all adversely affect thinking.

Overgrowth of yeast can create a buildup of *acetaldehyde* in the body. Yeast manufactures a little acetaldehyde as a by-product of its normal metabolism. Normally, we all have a little alcohol and acetaldehyde in our gut from everyday metabolism. But excess proliferation of yeast causes an increase in both. Elevated levels of acetaldehyde contribute to brain fog because it makes by-products that inhibit chemical messengers in the brain called neurotransmitters. Neurotransmitters that don't communicate well with each other can produce poor short-term memory, learning difficulties, and agitation.

Elevated levels of acetaldehyde can also produce severe fatigue. Acetaldehyde decreases the amount of oxygen available to tissues so you can get fatigued easily—

exercise is harder to perform, and healing is slower. It also decreases the availability of acetyl-CoA, which activates the citric acid cycle, the pathway that makes energy. In addition, acetaldehyde competes with vitamin B_6 and can adversely affect calcium and magnesium as well as irritate the lining of the intestinal tract.

What's the good news? The good news is that changing your diet and taking specific nutrients can decrease acetaldehyde.

Two-Month Program for CRC

This program includes a special diet along with nutrients and herbs. The diet and program are strict the first month and moderate the second. After that be more lenient. The diet is designed to avoid food items that promote yeast overgrowth: It is basically a low-carbohydrate, low *yeasty*-food diet.

However, the strictness of the diet is variable, because people have varying degrees of candidiasis. Mild cases need less strict diets and more severe cases need stricter ones. Some people require more stringent guidelines not because of their yeast problem, but because of other problems, such as inadequate digestive enzymes, inadequate specific nutrients, parasites, or food allergies. Over the years I saw many patients who, after doing a detoxification and rebuilding program, rid themselves of the yeast more quickly while eating a less strict diet.

Some doctors like to treat CRC with a medication called Diflucan for two weeks, followed by herbal and dietary methods. They say this shortens treatment time dramatically.

Dietary Suggestions for CRC

First Month:

Note: Spices may have mold on their leaves. If you have a mild problem you can still have some spices and even herbal tea if you pour boiling water over the leaves. Severe cases may need to avoid all leafy spices and herbal teas. Spices like curry and cinnamon cause fewer problems.

- Cut out all fruit. Mild cases can have a half a piece or small serving of fruit a day.
- Strictly avoid refined sugars, sucrose, fructose, dextrose, honey, maple syrup, barley malt, milk products containing milk sugar, alcohol, sweet potatoes, candies, caffeine, nuts, and pickled foods.
- Avoid yeast and fermented food items: mushrooms, cheeses, and vinegar don't cause yeast to grow, but if you have candidiasis you usually have mold sensitivities and this cross-reacts with other family food members—Brewers', bakers', and nutritional yeast; breads containing yeast; and soy sauce. Avoid pickled or smoked food products.
- Potatoes are okay for mild and moderate cases in moderate amounts but may make severe cases worse.
- Eliminate mildew in the home and mold on food. Do not eat cooked food that is more than two days old, or canned juices.

You can see how individualized this needs to be. Streamline your diet to your personal needs. If you get frustrated, check out Dr. Crook's book, *The Yeast Connection;* Sally Rockwell's *Coping with Candida Cookbook; The Yeast Syndrome* by Trowbridge and Walker; and Dr. Leo Galland's *The Four Pillars of Health.*

Second Month:
You can add one piece of fruit once a day or two halves at different times. Acidic fruits like berries, peaches, apricots, or citrus are usually well tolerated. You can also add more carbohydrate foods, but don't overdo it. Try to vary your food as much as possible so that you are not repeating the same food choices daily.

What *Can* You Eat?

Protein. Fish, organic meats (chicken, beef, turkey, duck), seafood of all kinds, eggs, goat, rabbit, lamb, venison, and other wild meats. Some individuals can handle soy products like tofu, or soy powder; others cannot.

Most vegetables except potatoes (but small potatoes are okay for mild cases).

Seeds and nuts in mild and moderate cases.

Grains, rotated. Try whole oats, rye, quinoa, millet, buckwheat, kamut, and amaranth. Amaranth is a seed-related grain, not a grass one, so even some severe cases of candidiasis may be able to tolerate this. Your health-food store should have products made from amaranth. Some severe cases need to avoid grains for a while.

Treats. Nibble on turkey or chicken or protein shakes (protein powder blended with nonsweetened soy or rice milk). Some people can handle popcorn with olive oil and garlic, soy nuts, and mochi heated and stuffed with tofu, chicken, turkey, or fish. (Mochi, available at health-food stores, is a compressed rice product. When toasted, it puffs up and can be stuffed or eaten as rice bread.) Others can tolerate berries with a little soy milk.

Typical Diet

Breakfast: Bowl of slow-cooked oats with butter and cinnamon, or whole-grain cereal with ground-up raw seeds and nuts and soy milk. Try some unleavened sprouted bread heated with a little butter. If you are severely reactive, you may not be able to tolerate this. Try it and see. If you don't seem to fare well with carbohydrates for breakfast, cook omelets or try foods like organic turkey in corn tortillas, turkey sausage, or protein shakes.

Lunch: Raw salad, beans, or protein (like organic chicken); whole-grain nonwheat crackers. Or soup and salad.

Dinner: Brown rice (if you can handle carbs); steamed or stirred veggies made with either tofu, organic chicken, turkey, or eggs and garlic, olive oil, and pieces of avocado.

Helpful Foods to Eat with Yeast Problems

"Safe" Potato Boats. Bake potatoes, scoop out much of insides, refill with stir-fried veggies. Can also mix with eggs or beans. Serve with diced scallions on top.

Dark leafy greens such as kale or chard. Stir-fry with equal parts of olive oil and water and a little butter.

Garlic. Use it to season all food generously, or cut a whole bulb in half, bake (in closed container or foil, or in open container covered with olive oil), and serve on yeast-free crackers.

Broccoli. Steam whole and serve with olive oil. Cut into fine pieces for salad. Steam and blend with butter to make broccoli soup.

Cauliflower. Serve same as broccoli or together.

Brussels sprouts. Steam well, chop into pieces, and eat with olive oil, salt and pepper. Or sauté with diced onions and zucchini, and serve over brown rice.

Tofu. Can usually be tolerated by mild and moderate cases, and by some, but not all, severe cases. Broil, then cut up into soups and veggie or grain dishes, or sauté in olive oil and serve with lettuce, tomato, and seasonings in a sandwich or corn tortilla.

Four Easy Home Soups

Green Soup Sauté spinach in a pan with olive oil, a little water, and lemon juice. Blend well. Add a little more water or lemon and seasonings.

Japanese Soup Put 5 tablespoons of miso in two quarts of water (play around with amount to taste). Bring to a boil. Add cut-up scallions, small pieces of broccoli, tofu (optional), and a package of mung-bean noodles, and cook five to ten minutes. Then add spinach leaves and pieces of your favorite fish, cooking at least another five minutes. If you cannot handle miso, make the soup with stock saved from steaming vegetables.

Red Fish Soup Sauté and then blend tomatoes, onions, garlic, green pepper, celery, and dark leafy greens. Put in soup pot. Heat well. Add mung-bean noodles. Five minutes before serving, add in fish pieces. You can use all kinds, from whitefish to shellfish.

Red Chicken Soup Same as Red Fish Soup, but add pieces of chicken.

Three Easy Juices

Tomato Spice Juice tomatoes, then add to taste some garlic, onions, celery, spinach leaves.

Green Cooler Juice cucumbers, celery, parsley, and a slice of apple.

Spicy High Roller Juice several inches of ginger, a little apple, half an orange, several stalks of celery, and a half to whole cucumber, depending on taste.

Healing Tea

Put one-fifth of a dropper of liquid extracts of each of the following into a pot of water: yellow dock, milk thistle and several drops of Pau D'Arco, and goldenseal. Heat gently, do not boil. Sip throughout the day.

Nutrients for CRC

After you have been on the diet for one week, start to add the supplements and herbs. When you do things in this order, you get fewer side effects. When you eradicate candida organisms, you have "dead" organisms traveling inside your body before they are eliminated (*die-off* or a *Herxheimer* reaction). You can get flu-like symptoms, fevers, aches, an increase of any of your past symptoms, etc., for a short period of time. Going on a restrictive diet first, before taking the nutrients, eliminates or lessens die-off symptoms in most people.

Nutrients for CRC (Six-Week Program)

(Add one new supplement a day)

- *Biotin.* 300 mcg three times a day prevents conversion of yeast into its more invasive fungal form.
- *Olive oil.* 2 teaspoons, to prevent spread of mycelia form of yeast.
- *Vitamin A.* 5,000 IU once a day.
- *Beta-carotene.* 5000 IU once a day.
- *Vitamin E.* 400 IU once a day.
- *Vitamin C.* 1 to 3 grams, divided dosages, throughout the day.
- *Vitamin B$_6$.* 30 to 50 mg once a day.
- *Magnesium.* 250 mg twice a day.
- *Glutamine.* 1 gram twice a day.
- *Essential fatty acids (EPA and evening primrose oil).* 3 capsules two to three times a day.
- *Oregano oil.* 6 to 10 drops in a capsule with meals, twice daily for six weeks.
- *Folic acid.* 400 mcg twice a day.
- *Zinc.* 20 mg a day and balance with 2 mg copper.
- *Glutathione.* 25 to 50 mg once a day.
- *Grapefruit-seed extract* products several times a day.
- *Probiotics mixtures.* 2 to 4 capsules three to four times a day. Take for two months, then twice a day for two more months.

Also consider: Products containing caprylic acid and commercial antifungal formulas available at health-food stores.

If you have had a lot of digestive symptoms, try nutrients in liquid form the first few months.

B complex vitamins. Use ones that are yeast free and hypoallergenic. Take them only every other day, since yeast can grow on B vitamins. Some severe cases of CRC cannot handle B vitamins until they get better. In this case, consume adequate amounts of raw seeds and whole grains like rice, oats, buckwheat, and millet, as well as plenty of fresh vegetables.

Vitamin C. If you are allergic to corn, get a hypoallergenic form, such as that made from sago palm.

Digestive enzymes. Low stomach acid may enhance yeast problems (see chapter 19). Stomach acid is a natural fungacidal agent, so insufficient stomach acid can complicate and prolong CRC as well as contribute to inadequate nutrient absorption, which can also lengthen healing time.

Natural anti-inflammatories. For the first month, consider several hundred mgs of bioflavonoids on an empty stomach several times a day. Circulating toxins from CRC can cause inflammation, and enzymes on an empty stomach act as anti-inflammatories. *Don't take them if you have active ulcers.*

Optional: For more energy you may consider adding several adrenal capsules and pantothenic acid, 500 mg three times daily. See resource section (appendix B) for products.

Helpful Herbs

The most helpful active agents are oregano, which contains multiple ingredients that act to combat bacteria, viruses, parasites, and fungi, and extract of goldenseal root (hydrastine). Oregano is such an effective natural antibiotic that you must be sure to take probiotics during treatment and especially afterward to rebuild the friendly bacteria of the intestinal tract.

Also useful are herbs that contain berberine (this is an alkaloid found in the berberica botanical family, which includes goldenseal, Oregon grape, barberry, and Pau D'Arco). Other beneficial products may be urva ursi, and tea tree or olive-leaf oils. Sage and rosemary in oil forms contain eucalyptus oil, which destroys *Candida albicans*, worms, and harmful bacteria. Healing with herbs unfortunately is a trial-and-error method, and, since there are so many strains of candida, some people respond better to certain botanicals than others. However, oil of oregano seems to help many sufferers with CRC.

Pau D'Arco bark bath. Place 3 tablespoon of Pau D'Arco tea leaves in cheesecloth and tie over the faucet where the water comes into the tub, so that the water flows through the tea. In essence, you are making a tub of tea. This is especially helpful for difficult cases. One young boy had severe behavior problems due to CRC. His mother had a difficult time getting him to change his diet. Once he began the Pau D'Arco baths, he calmed down enough to cooperate with the diet and his healing skyrocketed.

Yeast and Disease

Research in the Scandinavian *Journal of Gastroenterology* studied 19 patients with *inflammatory bowel disease* of the Crohn's type. One month they ate their normal diet. The second month they followed a low-yeast diet (excluding vine-gar, alcohol, breads, malted cereals, dairy products, B vitamins from yeast sources, and refined sugar and flour). The disease was much less active while on the low-yeast diet, as measured by a Crohn's disease activity index (CDAI). This, as well as other studies, suggests that *dietary yeast and/or the candida-related complex may possibly contribute to inflammatory bowel conditions.*

For resistant cases of *herpes*, try a candida program for four weeks. Con-comitant infections with both can resist healing until both are treated.

Mind-Body Techniques

Reflex Points

On the feet, work all the intestinal points from the stomach to the rectal points around the heel. Find tender points and hold them. Then very firmly rub the entire sole of each foot and around both ankles with your knuckles. (See foot reflexology charts at the end of chapter 20.)

17 The Intestinal Tract and Serious Disease: Colorectal Cancer and AIDS

The health of the intestinal tract can play a role in any disease, as it affects whole-body nutrition, immunity, and vitality. Two important diseases that are related to the health of the intestinal tract are cancer of the colon and rectum, and AIDS.

Colorectal Cancer (Cancer of the Colon and the Rectum)

Cancers of the colon and rectum are some of the most prevalent cancers and leading causes of death in the Western world. They are life-threatening diseases that require medical supervision. It is mentioned here basically in regard to preventing the disease.

Colorectal cancer is a slow-growing disease that has usually gone on for a long time before there are any symptoms, such as bleeding, fatigue, or pain. It is an epithelial cancer, meaning the cancer arises out of the epithelial layer—cells that line the intestinal tract. It is thought to be a progressive disease that involves uncontrolled growth (hyperproliferation) of this epithelial lining, which can then directly lead to cancer, or to polyps (wartlike growths or offshoots of the epithelium). Over time, as an untreated polyp stays in the colon, the risk for colon cancer increases. If a polyp is one centimeter or larger and has been in the colon for five years, the risk of developing colon cancer is 2.5 percent higher; after ten years in the colon, it is 8 percent higher, and after 20 years it is 24 percent higher than in people who do not have polyps.

The incidence of colon cancer has been rising in North America, especially in African Americans. At higher risk, also, are those of Jewish descent. In countries closer to the equator and in Finland there is a much lower rate of this cancer, but the incidence increases when people from these countries move to higher-risk areas. This points a finger to elements in the environment, such as diet, as increasing this risk. Colorectal cancer used to be less frequent in Japan than in the Western world, but it has been increasing there, which is thought to be due to increased consumption of total fat and saturated fat.

Diets of Western countries (high in junk foods and deficient in healthy foods) have been shown to promote uncontrolled growth of epithelial tissues, which, along with genetic factors, may increase the risk of colorectal cancer.

To Decrease Your Risk of Getting Colorectal Cancer

Fiber. The understanding of the role of dietary fiber as a protector against colorectal cancer has flip-flopped over the past several decades. Since the 1950s and 1960s, fiber has been thought to protect against this cancer. A recent study from Harvard on women did not support this protective effect. However, what was considered to be a high-fiber diet, based on American intake, may not have been comparable to the amount of fiber consumed in countries where there is less colon cancer, so the outcome of the Harvard study may be clouded. There have also been numerous studies that demonstrate the *beneficial* effect of fiber, such as the 1997 study led by Martha L. Slattery, which showed that a diet higher in fiber decreased the risk of colon cancer in older men and women, while a diet higher in refined grains (less fiber) was associated with more colon cancer. So to say that it has been proven that fiber is not protective against colorectal cancer is inaccurate.

High-fiber foods are thought to be protective against colon cancer for a number of reasons:

1. Fiber is acted upon by friendly bacteria to make protective, anticancer substances.
2. A diet low in fiber takes two to three times as long to transit through the intestinal tract. In a sluggish intestine, unfriendly colonic bacteria—higher in the colons of people who eat less fiber—have more opportunity to break down normal bile acid in the intestines (which help digest fats) into cancer-causing substances. Societies with less colon cancer have an average bowel transit time of 20 to 24 hours—almost half the time as in Western cultures. (See chapter 1 to learn how to easily check your transit time.)
3. The phytic acid in grains is thought to be an active and protective agent in reducing the risk of cancer in the colon.
4. Fiber-rich foods act as fuel for short-chain fatty acids that protect the lining of the intestinal tract.

In other words, *keep eating whole grains, veggies, fruits, seeds, and nuts along with your protein choices.* Fiber is still a good thing.

Selenium. Lower blood levels of selenium have been associated with higher rates of polyp formation. One study demonstrated that the lowest selenium blood levels were associated with the most advanced disease states (although whether this is the chicken or the egg is hard to tell). Selenium may be a promising agent in preventing colon cancer by enhancing blood levels of an enzyme called glutathione peroxidase, which is protective of the intestines.

Dietary Fat. The link between how much and what kind of fat we eat and colorectal cancer has a controversial history. Some studies suggest that we are more at risk of getting colorectal cancer the more we eat fat, especially saturated fat from animals. Consuming fish oils has been shown to decrease risk, which may be why the fish-eating Japanese and Greenland Inuits have lower incidences of colorectal cancer. Yet, a combined analysis of thirteen studies suggested that the type of fat we eat does not make a difference. Like fiber, the results of studies on fat and colon cancer zigzag. Certain isolated studies suggest that coconut oil, olive oil, and safflower oil enhance tumor growth while fish oil does not. A study of cancer trends and diet in fifteen Euorpean countries did not show a consistant pattern.

What to do? Be sensible. Attempt to cut down on fats in general and animal fats in particular, and eat more fruits and vegetables. *It is probably more the methods used to cook meats and fish, which contain fat, more than the fats themselves,* that play the most influential role in getting colorectal cancer.

How you cook makes a difference. Heterocyclic amines (HCA) are *mutagens* (cause alterations in genetic material leading to more risk of cancer) and *carcinogens* (substances known to cause cancer) and have been found to cause tumors in animals. HCAs are formed when meat and fish are very well cooked or cooked at very high temperatures, such as when barbecuing or frying, and turn dark brown at the surfaces (this does not include blackening from spices, which is different than dark surfaces from high temperature cooking). HCAs are more present in red meat and chicken than in fish, and are not present in meats and fish that are stewed, baked, or microwaved.

The most prevalent HCA in the American diet associated with an increased risk of colon cancer is called *PhIP.* It is found in high amounts in fried and barbecued chicken. In a study that looked at the cooking methods, meat intake, and polyp formation of hundreds of people, it was found that people who ate more red meat and more fried red meat got more precancerous polyps. The study showed that eating red meat more than once a week, frying it more than 10 percent of the time, and consuming the meat with a dark brown surface from the cooking doubled the risk of getting colon cancer.

Note: HCAs are *not* formed in vegetables, as it is the fat in meats, together with heat, that forms them.

Cooked milk protein (casein) which causes abrasion of the intestinal wall, has been shown to promote colon cancer in animals. It is thought to be harder to digest than uncooked casein. This is hypothesized to be a factor contributing to uncontrolled growth of intestinal tissue. Avoid daily consumption of *cooked cheeses* (like those on pizza and in casseroles) and get into the habit of substituting soy or nut milks for regular milk and cream in recipes for baked goods.

On the other hand, "fat-free" dairy products may protect against colon cancer. Fat-free or skim milk contains several sphingolipids, substances that protect against colon cancer. Animal studies even suggest these substances reverse precancerous changes. So if you eat dairy, consume nonfat milk and cheeses.

Calcium and vitamin D. Remember that colon cancer is an epithelial cancer, meaning the polyps and cancer arise out of the epithelial layer of the intestinal tract. A Western-type diet has been found to produce excess growth of epithelial cells in the intestinal tract, which may contribute to increased risk for polyps and colon cancer. Calcium and vitamin D have both been shown to markedly suppress hyperproliferation of tissues in the colon. Calcium may do this by binding to the irritating fatty acids in foods and inactivating them. *So take your calcium supplements with meals.* Also, the risk of large bowel cancer, especially rectal cancer, has been shown to decrease by increasing blood levels of metabolites (breakdown products) of vitamin D.

Helpful nutrients. Thiamin, vitamin B_6, and folic acid seem to be protective agents, especially in people with a family history of colorectal cancer. In fact, high dosages of folic acid, which need to be administered by a physician, have even been used to reduce some symptoms of advanced colorectal cancer such as serious diarrhea.

Friendly bacteria. It has been suggested that an altered colonic environment may predispose some of us to colorectal cancer. Make sure your diet contains adequate fiber so friendly bacteria will thrive. Consume cultured products such as yogurt, fermented foods like sauerkraut, and pickled foods like beets, beans, or okra several times a week, or take friendly bacterial supplements (probiotics) such as *Bifidobacteria,* which lower the accumulation of the toxic *Clostridium* species that has been linked to colon cancer.

Alcohol and smoking. Alcohol has been consistently shown to increase the risk of precancerous polyp formation. In one California study it was shown that consuming alcohol on a daily basis doubled the risk of colorectal cancer. Alcohol may affect bile composition, irritate intestinal lining, cause uncontrolled intestinal tissue growth, and alter hormonal signaling. Eliminate alcohol abuse. Smoking has been shown to be a risk factor in some studies, particularly with men. Current smoking influences the risk most, so stop smoking.

Job-related substances. People who work with asbestos and cement have been found to have an increased incidence of cancer in the right side of the colon. The folks who work with these materials should heed protective advice and avoid risk factors as much as possible, and certainly more rigorously if colon cancer runs in their families.

Once you have colon cancer, if it goes untreated, it usually progresses rapidly and causes death. However, Edward Leyton, M.D., reported the case of one of his patients who refused surgery, chemotherapy, or radiation. This sixty-two-year-old man began a vegan diet (animal free), emphasizing vegetables, fruits, whole grains, and legumes along with nutrient supplements. He lived well beyond his expected survival time and was healthier than before (he was sixty-seven years old at the time the case was reported). This in no way means you should refuse orthodox treatment. However, it emphasizes that how you live and eat can make a huge difference, not only in prevention but also in quality of life once you have a diagnosis of colorectal cancer. Do not rely only on surgery, radiation, or chemotherapy. Nutrition is a primary component of digestive health.

If you have a history of colon polyps, or if colon cancer runs in your family:

- Eat fish and take *fish oil* supplements (2 to 5 capsules twice a day).
- Avoid fried and barbecued meats.
- Avoid cooking cheese and consume fat-free dairy products.
- Drink *green tea*. It protects against all kinds of cancers and, when consumed together with whole grains in the diet, is particularly protective against colon cancer.
- Consume *dark green leafy veggies* several times a week. Eat lots of colored veggies and fruits daily (some raw).
- Take *calcium* (500 mg or more) and *vitamin D supplements* (40 to 500 IU daily; higher levels for people with active colorectal cancer), *with* meals.
- Take B_{12}, B_6, and *folic acid*.
- Take 150 mcg of *selenium* daily.
- Take an *antioxidant formula* once or twice a day.
- Take *Bifidobacteria* (three billion organisms daily).
- Avoid smoking and daily alcohol.
- Spend at least 15 to 20 minutes outdoors daily.
- Do digestive exercises and meditations several times a week.

A Note about Stomach and Esophageal Cancer

Esophageal cancer has been found to be higher in people with symptomatic heartburn. Implicated is not the heartburn, but the treatment. Drugs to suppress acid secretion are so effective that the body responds by increasing (hyperproliferating) the secreting cells.

Human and animal studies suggest that a deficiency in stomach acid, and hyperproliferation of cells in these tissues, increases the risk of getting cancer of the stomach and esophagus. These studies raise concerns about prolonged use of acid suppressant therapies, meaning *don't abuse antacids* (see chapter 6 for information on other ways to treat esophageal reflux).

In one study, 228 patients with stomach cancer were compared to patients without gatrointestinal disease. The biggest difference was that patients without cancer ate many more raw vegetables, especially uncooked lettuce, tomatoes, carrots, coleslaw, and red cabbage. So eat your salads!

AIDS

AIDS is an extremely complicated disease that requires intensive medical supervision. This short section on AIDS is included because the intestinal tract plays a number of pivotal roles in the disease, especially in the risk factors for a compromised immune system. Usually it is problems with the intestinal tract that lead to the initial clinical diagnosis of AIDS. For example, a parasite infection or a cancer of the digestive tract can be the first presenting sign of AIDS. Also, most AIDS patients exhibit gastrointestinal symptoms at some time during the course of the disease. The following information is meant to contribute to a dialogue between the AIDS patient and his or her doctor.

Parasites and the Immune System

Not everyone exposed to the AIDS virus gets the disease AIDS. This is a critical fact because it indicates the existence of risk factors that play a role in determining how vulnerable someone is to this disease. This suggests that the probability of getting AIDS may be decreased by reducing risk factors, both in those who are not yet infected and in those who carry the virus but do not have the outright disease. It is thought that a compromised immune system is one of the ways in which a person becomes vulnerable to getting AIDS. The health of the intestinal environment plays a vital role in determining a person's overall immune competency.

One prominent risk factor that may compromise a person's immune system is parasitic infection. Scientists are presently theorizing that before the AIDS epidemic took off, it was preceded by an epidemic of intestinal parasitic infections that spread through sexual transmission. The infections depressed the immune system in many gay men, making them more vulnerable to the AIDS virus. Intestinal parasites are also thought to contribute to the ongoing spread of AIDS. Many of these parasitic infections go undetected, as there may be no symptoms, or only minor ones. Nonetheless, parasites may be passed on to lovers through sex and to friends or roommates through contact with food and household objects.

How Parasitic Infections Can Suppress Immunity

- As parasites burrow into the intestinal lining, they directly damage the intestinal wall, which disrupts the intestinal environment.

- Parasites give off toxins that can further damage the wall.
- A damaged intestinal wall is more permeable, allowing the AIDS virus more free access to the bloodstream through the numerous capillaries within the gut wall.
- All this can inflame the intestinal wall and contribute to malabsorption, which can then make even a quality diet hard to digest. In turn, this results in malnutrition. All these elements further weaken the immune system.
- Parasites stimulate T helper cells, which increase the multiplication of the AIDS virus within cells.

All high-risk individuals, as well as their sexual partners, should be tested for parasites, treated together, and retested once a year as recurrence with these infections is high. It is important to use labs and methods with the highest chance of picking up an infection. (Check appendix B for the list of labs known to do thorough workups on parasites.) Ask about test methods that require a purge technique (you drink something that purges your intestines, which encourages parasites embedded in the gut wall to loosen). Sometimes one test will not reveal parasites while another may, so repeat testing is to be considered when symptoms persist but parasites have not yet been detected.

It is also essential to work with a physician who appreciates that some non-pathogenic intestinal bugs (meaning ones that are not known to cause *obvious* disease) may be risk factors. These nonpathogenic bugs can indicate that a parasitic infection is present but has not yet been found. Some doctors treat for these agents and some do not. I think it is a good idea to consider these as warning signals and do some sort of intervention.

People with HIV disease and AIDS should be very careful about which drugs they take to treat parasites, and should work with a physician to construct individualized programs. See chapter 15 for symptoms and treatment of parasites. Discuss these suggestions with the doctors who know your case.

Patients with AIDS tend to have two clinical patterns of parasitic infections depending on the level of their immune competence (identified by CD4+ T-cell count levels). A better-preserved immune system usually means the infection will respond to treatment, while those with more impaired immune systems usually tend toward persistent infections with chronic watery diarrhea, malabsorption, and weight loss. In either case, rebuilding the intestinal tract with the nutrients mentioned in this section is helpful. Also, since malabsorption and malnutrition can cause a weakened immune system, read the chapters on digestive tools and review the deficiency charts to see if you have a number of signs indicating low tissue levels of specific vital nutrients (page 11).

Diarrhea and AIDS

Diarrhea is a complication in 60 percent of patients with AIDS. Chronic diarrhea depletes the body of strength and nutrients and needs to be addressed for maintaining health.

Mild diarrhea (less than four unformed bowel movements a day) usually can be treated with friendly bacteria (probiotics in supplement form as well as yogurt), bananas, applesauce, fruit cocktail, Citrucel (ground-up citrus peels, which can be less gassy than psyllium fiber) or some other fiber source (see fiber cocktail, page 25), 1 to 5 grams of glutamine throughout the day, along with high dosages of folic acid (1 to 5 mgs), zinc (20 mg twice a day) and vitamin B complex.

Diarrhea that is more severe should be treated by your doctor, who may suggest an appropriate antibiotic.

To help with more severe cases of diarrhea, for six weeks take:

- 6 to 10 drops of *oil of oregano* in gelatin capsules, twice a day, 5 minutes after meals.
- 1 to 5 grams of *glutamine* spread throughout the day.
- 1 to 5 mgs a day of *folic acid.*
- 20 mg of *zinc* twice a day.
- *Probiotic supplements* and *yogurt.*
- 2 *garlic tablets* with meals three times a day.
- *Buffered vitamin* C. Several grams throughout the day with *bioflavonoids.*
- *Vitamin B complex* (yeast free). 100 mg one to three times a day.

Complications of AIDS are often treated with antibiotics, and *C. difficile* diarrhea may be caused by taking antibiotics like ampicillin/amoxicillin, cephalosporins (like Keflex), or clindamycin (Cleocin). Of note, one study identified clindamycin use and prolonged hospitalization as the main risk factors for *C. difficile* infections in AIDS patients. You can try to treat this kind of diarrhea with a yeast called *Saccharomyces boulardii,* which can be purchased at healthfood stores. If this doesn't work, Mark Bowers, writing for the Bulletin of Experimental Treatments for AIDS, warns that this kind of diarrhea should only be treated with metronidazole. (If alcohol has been consumed within 24 hours of taking this antibiotic, it can cause severe vomiting. Ritonavir contains alchohol and AIDS patients taking ritonavir should not be given metronidazole.)

There are many opportunistic organisms that can thrive in the immune-suppressed AIDS patient. Infections with *Cryptosporidium parvum* are quite common. The first line of treatment to discuss with your doctor is Humatin, along with colostrum, antifungals (like oil of oregano, pharmacueticals, or both), garlic, and the other products mentioned above. Cryptosporidial diarrhea that doesn't respond to this first line of treatment can become severe and chronic.

Bowers says that an increasing cause of diarrhea in AIDS patients are two species of parasites called *Enterocytozoon bieneusi* and *Septata intestinalis*. Albendazole at 200 to 400 mg twice a day for one month is promising for *S. intestinalis*. Somewhat helpful for those with *E. bieneusi* is a low-fat, low-fiber diet with simple carbohydrates. Review all recommendations with your doctor. His Web site (www.sfaf.org/treatment/beta/b33dia.html) is a very helpful source of information about possible intestinal infections and what can be done about them.

Other Factors

Deficiencies in the digestive enzymes—stomach acid, pancreatic enzymes, and sometimes even bile—can contribute to or worsen bouts of diarrhea, so read the chapter on digestive tools and see if these are helpful. Since common bacterial pathogens may cause more problems in AIDS patients than in those without the disease, taking digestive supplements along with nutrients mentioned below may be helpful for AIDS patients.

AIDS also reduces the ability of the digestive tract to digest nutrients, and this condition gets worse as the disease progresses. Consider intravenous vitamin infusions, B_{12} injections, and liquid nutrients to optimize tissue levels and keep the immune system functioning better. The various digestive exercises, affirmations, and meditations at the end of different chapters in this book can be added into your regime several times a week.

Six-Week Protective Intestinal Regime for AIDS

- *Oil of oregano.* 6 to 10 drops in gelatin capsules twice a day with meals.
- *Glutamine.* 1,000 mg, three to five times a day.
- *Zinc.* 20 mg, 1 to 2 times a day.
- *Probitoics* 2 to 4 capsules two to four times a day.
- *Yogurt and cultured foods* consumed generously.
- *Fiber cocktail* once a day (see chapter 2) and consume unprocessed whole foods.
- *B vitamin complex,* including extra folic acid, B_{12}, and B_6 (consider B_{12} injection or sublingual B_{12}).
- *Vitamin A.* 25,000 IU daily. (Ask your doctor)
- *Selenium.* 200 mcg daily.
- *Proteolytic enzymes.* 6 between meals twice a day to aid digestion and combat inflammation and free radicals.

- *Digestive enzymes* with meals to assist in digestion and reduce allergic or intolerant food reactions.
- *Multiple vitamin/mineral supplements* in liquid form

Sensible Maintenance Tips

- *Testosterone levels.* Get baseline and monitor every six months, watching for decline, which could mean you're losing muscle mass.
- *Resistance exercise,* like weight lifting (even if very low weight or just pushing against a wall) four times a week. (Daily exercise regimes may stress the immune system.)
- *Weight check* weekly.
- *Triglyceride levels* should be monitored, as high levels suggest increased disease activity in asymptomatic AIDS patients or warn of secondary infections that require treatment. Can be caused by certain drugs, too.
- Consider amino acid blends, bovine colostrum, digestive affirmations, exercises, and meditiations.

Do intestinal protective program every six months as prevention as well as acute care. Check www.sfaf.org/treatment/betalive/b1297nut.html. There is a wealth of information online. Also check out *POZ* magazine, dedicated to latest info on AIDS.

Helpful Herbs

Milk thistle weed (silymarin), astragalus, a mushroom extract called somastatin, and hypericum have been reported to possibly inhibit retroviral infections.

PART III

How to Find Out What's Wrong and Fix It

Food Allergies
Digestive Enzymes
Detoxification and Rebuilding Program

18 Finding and Healing Your Food Allergies

Food allergies can cause, as well as aggravate, many digestive complaints. On the other hand, intestinal illnesses can cause food allergies. Thus, in a book on digestive problems, food allergies must be addressed. This chapter will help you understand how food allergies and digestive problems go hand in hand. The good news is that many (not all) food allergies, once identified and avoided while you improve your digestion and nutrition, can be reduced or eliminated.

However, get traditional doctors and holistic doctors together in a room to debate food allergies and you're apt to have a fight. The *concept* of food allergy is accepted by traditional doctors, but the fact that a food allergy might *cause* or *aggravate* digestive and other health problems isn't. Even though hard science supports the link between food allergies and many illnesses—such as gastrointestinal problems, ulcers, colitis, gallbladder problems, colic, headaches, and even learning disabilities—the role of food allergies in disease is minimized by mainstream medicine. Why?

First, the underlying mechanisms of food allergies are still not exactly understood, which makes food allergies unappreciated. Second, the medical establishment has historically been resistant to new ideas concerning the link between food and health, and this bias extends to food allergies.

All this arguing over what you have—whether it is an allergic reaction to food or a reaction to a food based on other mechanisms—is moot. You suffer anyway. And a significant number of chronic problems are often improved by figuring out food allergies and avoiding or rotating those foods.

Try it. Go on a one-week elimination diet and see what happens to your symptoms. Generally, if you feel a lot better after avoiding the foods you normally eat and consuming only foods that usually don't cause discomfort, you've got a pretty good idea that you've got food allergies, or whatever you want to call them. This chapter explains what is called the *allergy elimination-reintroduction* program.

DON, THE DOUBTING SCIENTIST

Don was a tall, thin genius who had severe bleeding colitis. He had been off and on steroids for years, but not only didn't they cure his colitis, they created other health problems. I told Don that milk allergies were a common aggravating factor for colitis. Don thought that if this were true, he would have been told so by his regular doctor. He ran a medical literature search anyway, and lo and behold, he found numerous scientific articles discussing the milk-colitis link. He gave up dairy products on the spot. He improved so much, he decided to read more and started to test himself for multiple foods. He discovered he had problems with tea, corn, carrots, onions, potatoes, and lettuce. Staying off his allergy foods kept his colitis quiet. Don was no longer doubting.

PANIC ATTACKS, HEART PALPITATIONS, AND FOOD ALLERGIES

An article in *The Lancet,* a British medical journal, called "Food Allergy: Fact or Fiction?" tells of a thirty-seven-year-old woman who had episodes of heart palpitations, breathing difficulties, and pain. She was diagnosed as having a pulmonary embolism (lung clot), and given drugs. She got better for a while and went off the medications. Then her mother died of a heart attack and the woman's symptoms returned, worse than before. She became depressed and fearful. She had to take a taxi even to go to work at her fruit shop, which was only 200 yards from her home, as she was too phobic to walk on the street. She'd become almost completely housebound. No disease could be found.

At this point she was referred to an allergy clinic at the department of medicine at the University of Liverpool. Foods were introduced through a tube in her nose so the woman would not know which foods were being tested. At the same time, she was hooked up to a heart monitor. Tea, coffee, and tomatoes reproduced her panic symptoms, as well as causing superventricular tachycardia (rapid heartbeat—160 heartbeats per minute). Avoiding these foods promptly got rid of her symptoms, and she was able to resume a normal life.

How Can Foods Cause Problems?

For certain sensitive people, food allergies are a common sources of intestinal problems —from gas and constipation to irritable bowel syndrome, inflammatory bowel disease, gallstones, and ulcers. The authors of the above *Lancet* article, Drs. Ronald Finn and H. Newman Cohen, made some enlightening statements about how food allergies might cause these problems. They wrote:

"This clinical study supports the view that *some foods may cause widespread and disabling symptoms in people who are sensitive to them. . . .* [italics mine] The

Research now shows that food can cause diseases, such as heart disease, high blood pressure, diabetes, gallbladder disease, and gastrointestinal disease. It also seems feasible that allergic responses to foods have the potential to cause disease.

offending agent (food allergy) is often a favorite food which is taken daily, usually in large quantities. The most likely possibility is that patients with food allergy have some degree of enzyme deficiency, which leads to difficulty in metabolizing certain foods; and it is the consequent build-up of intermediate metabolites which causes toxic symptoms."

Why Is the Incidence of Food Allergies Increasing?

There are a number of reasons:

- Untreated maldigestion and malabsorption burden the intestinal lining and disrupt the flora balance, contributing to food allergies and to the intestinal lining becoming extra permeable.
- You can be predisposed by inherited genes.
- A *Western lifestyle* has been linked to allergies, possibly because junk-food consumers are exposed to processed oils, refined foods, and excessive sugars that damage the intestinal lining and contribute to hypersensitive reactions to foods. And industrial pollution burdens the liver, which can contribute to food allergy problems.
- *H. pylori* infections are increasing and appear to be associated with food allergies, especially in children.
- Non-nursing mothers can expose their baby's immature immune system to foreign food molecules.
- *Emotional stress.* Never fail to appreciate the role of stress on the intestinal tract. I know numerous cases where patients spent thousands of dollars seeing specialists and got little relief, only to find when they reduced their stress (e.g., got a divorce) their chronic allergy symptoms went away. Reduce your stress levels any way you can.

Clues That You May Have Food Allergies

- *Chronic digestive problems.*
- *Recurring infections* of any kind (respiratory, sinusitis, kidney, urinary, tonsillitis, and ear).
- *Recurring inflammatory conditions* of any kind (gastrointestinal, joints, or vascular system).
- *Difficulty losing excess weight.*
- Unexplained bouts of *severe fatigue* after eating.
- *Tendency to hold water (edema)* that is not associated with the cyclic fluid retention of menstrual cycling—waking up with fingers swollen or knuckles whitish and stiff, face swollen, eyes puffy from an unexplained

cause, swelling in face or fingers within hours after eating, ankle swelling that is not due to a heart condition.

- *Chronic "allergic shiners"*—dark rings under or around your eyes that are not due to loss of sleep, illness, or pain.
- *Chronic horizontal creases under the lower eyelid,* almost looking as if your skin was "pinched," that may get worse after meals.
- *Frequent stuffy nose or postnasal drip* for no explainable reason, which may last for several hours after meals, or clearing your throat frequently after eating.
- *Chronically swollen glands,* with no known reason.
- Bouts of *anxiety, sweating, or heart palpitations* within several hours of eating.
- Frequent unexplained *skin rashes* (often a sign of allergy to sodium benzoate, yeast, aspirin, or related compounds).
- *Immediate family members with food allergies or asthma.*
- *History of gallbladder disease.*
- *History of acne.*
- *History of taking antibiotics.*
- *Mental "fuzziness" or "fogginess"* after eating.
- Bouts of *"low blood sugar"* that don't go away.
- *Headaches* that don't go away.
- *General ill feelings* that do not go away and are not explainable.

In children signs of possible food allergies are: persistent swollen glands, enlarged tonsils, recurring middle-ear infection, chronic fluid behind the eardrums, asthma, frequent temper tantrums, hyperactivity, frequent redness of the ears, or paleness or blotchiness of the face after eating. Also, pulling at the nose after eating or cranky and behavioral changes after eating may be suggestive. In 1959, *an exhaustive study showed 83 to 90 percent of bed-wetting was linked to food allergy.* The most common food culprit was milk. This study has been replicated.

Note: Helpful books on the subject include: *Solving the Puzzle of Your Hard-To-Raise Child* and *Tracking Down Hidden Food Allergy,* by Dr. William Crook, a pediatrician; *Is This Your Child?* by Dr. Doris Rapp, a pediatric allergist. Videos and books are available through Dr. Rapp's Practical Allergy Research Foundation, Tahoma Clinic Books, and Keats Publishing (see appendix B).

Helpful Hints for Sleuthing Out Your Food Allergies

1. Keep a one-week diet diary, noting everything you eat.
2. Note what foods you eat at least once a day. This can be tricky, as they may be added to other foods. For example, wheat is in bread, sauces, cookies, gravies, and pasta.

3. Write down your three favorite foods.
4. Note which foods on lists two and three overlap. Foods on both lists are *suspects*.

Why Do We Often Crave Foods We're Allergic To?

Studies have shown that eating foods to which we are allergic can elevate blood sugar in a way that is similar to consuming foods high in sugar. We actually get a sort of "high" from these foods, and that contributes to our desire to eat them.

Some allergy foods have protein-like substances that have opioid properties, meaning they can act like endorphins, molecules that make you feel exhilarated. Some foods contain natural morphine-like substances. Examples are wheat and milk proteins, which can act like opioids, or elevating mood substances. Milk and wheat opioids can bind with receptor sites in your brain, thereby contributing to a subtle sense of increased well-being. This is theorized to create an *addiction/craving* relationship with that particular food.

You might have heard some people say that once they start to eat carbohydrates (like bread) or sugars (like ice cream) they can't stop. But if they just sit tight and make it through abstinence from these foods for one to two weeks, the cravings stop. I think the opioid factor is largely responsible for this phenomenon. In this sense, we are actually addicted to certain foods. *Thus, our most suspicious foods for allergens are usually those we crave and eat the most often.*

Two Basic Types of Food Allergies

Immediate food allergies occur within minutes to hours after you eat a food. Because of this, it's fairly easy to tell what food is causing your reaction. This type of allergic reaction is also called an immediate hypersensitive reaction (meaning you immediately are overly sensitive to eating this food).

An immediate reaction involves immunoglobulin IgE. The reaction is usually permanent, meaning that either you are born with it or, once you develop it, it stays with you for the rest of your life. This type of allergic reaction is often reproducible, predictable, and severe. It usually affects the intestinal lining, causing diarrhea and bloating, as well as swelling of the eyes or lips and even the throat. However, only a *few* food allergies are immediate.

Delayed allergy reactions, or masked allergies, are the most common food-allergy reactions. They are called *masked* because these are not immediate reactions like the ones above, and the correlation between eating a food and the reaction to it is hidden. This reaction can happen from several hours to as long as four or five days after you eat the food, depending on your intestinal-transit time. As long as a food is in you, it can cause an allergic reaction.

For example, if you were allergic to beef and ate a hamburger on Saturday night, if you have a slow intestinal-transit time (see chapter 1), you may not experience allergic symptoms, like abdominal discomfort, until Monday. Do you see how delayed food reactions can be confusing? The relationship to the beef on Saturday and the symptom (pain) on Monday is *masked*. The reaction is several days later, and it's hard to connect eating the hamburger with *causing* the bellyache.

Delayed food reactions, which are rarely life threatening, may cause various reactions throughout the body. Sometimes delayed reactions are dependent on how much food you eat. You may not react to a little food, whereas eating a lot of that food may cause a problem. The promising news is that with temporary avoidance, along with the use of digestive aids and rebuilding the intestinal and body vitality, a number of *delayed* food reactions may be diminished or eliminated over time.

The Allergy Elimination Diet

An *allergy elimination-reintroduction diet* consists of avoiding foods and then reintroducing them in a specific way to test your reactions to them. The diet is maintained for one week, ten days, or two weeks, however long it takes for all your symptoms to go away.

This not only helps you identify food allergies, but will also give you a strong understanding about your body's relationship to particular foods and how your body, when stressed, reacts. This is valuable information that makes a person *body-wise.*

Read labels. Foods can be hidden inside other foods. For example, some rice and soy milks have added corn or safflower oils and malt sweeteners. Make sure there are no hidden allergens, such as casein and whey (dairy products). Check your vitamins, too.

The Elimination Diet—Foods to Avoid

Foods you eat more than three times a week or any foods you suspect along with the following.

Dairy products: milk, cheese, butter, cottage cheese, yogurt, ice cream; also whey, casein, sodium caseinate, calcium caseinate, and any foods that have these in them.

Wheat: most breads, pastas, pastries, cookies, cakes, numerous gravies, and foods that contain wheat, as well as durum semolina and farina.

Soy: soy sauce, miso, soy milk, tofu, tempeh, soy isolates, and foods like soy protein powders.

Corn: corn chips, corn on the cob, foods with added corn as well as foods that contain corn products such as corn oil, corn syrup, corn sweetener, dextrose and glucose (they are corn-derived), or foods containing unspecified vegetable oil.

Yeast: avoid all vitamin supplements or foods with yeast (such as baked goods) or brewers' yeast, like many processed herbs and spices.

Beef and pork: hamburgers, steaks, bacon, chops, or any foods that contain them, such as soups.

Eggs: both egg yolks and whites, and foods that contain them, such as mayonnaise.

Citrus: lemons, oranges, grapefruits, tangerines, mandarin oranges, limes, and any foods containing them, such as citrus herbal teas.

Carrots, apples, and berries. Allergies can occur to vegetables and fruit, the most common being to carrots and apples. Other frequent ones are lettuce, potatoes, onions, tomatoes, and garlic. (It is hard to know if you are having a reaction to the pesticides or the actual food, so you may want to try eating organic fruits and vegetables.)

Coffee and tea: no caffeinated or decaffeinated coffee or tea unless it is herbal and does not contain citrus.

Peanuts and peanut butter are also a common allergen.

Alcohol.

Refined sugars: Avoid all table sugar or any foods that contain it (such as candy, pies, cookies, chewing gum, chocolate bars), cane sweeteners, fructose, sucrose, glucose, dextrose, corn sweeteners, corn syrups, maltose, and levulose; artificial sweeteners.

Processed oils, hydrogenated oils, artificial colors or flavors, preservatives, additives.

Tap water: Use only spring, distilled, or filtered water that comes in glass or heavy plastic containers. Cook with this water and carry it with you wherever you go, including to restaurants.

The Elimination Diet—Foods You Can Eat

Grains: rice, millet, oats, quinoa, amaranth, kamut, spelt, and buckwheat in whole grain, pasta, or cereal form without oils, fruits, eggs, sugars, or wheat added. May use rice, almond, or oat milk on cereals (or water with a little white grape juice added for flavor).

Proteins: chicken, turkey (unprocessed in any way), lamb, rabbit, duck, and fish, except for shellfish like shrimp, lobster, and scallops. Canned tuna, salmon, and sardines are fine if packed in spring water.

Legumes: beans that are usually okay to eat for protein are lentils, string beans, red, black, and kidney beans, garbanzos, split peas, Kentucky wonders, mung beans, and any beans other than soy. (Soak overnight and pour off the water, rinse and add more water before cooking.) You can eat bean soups and dips but be careful of added sugars, etc.

However, if you are a vegetarian and normally eat grains, beans, and nuts, you may want to avoid the ones you most commonly consume to identify which are your allergens.

Vegetables: All vegetables except corn, lettuce, potatoes, onions, tomatoes, garlic, and carrots.

Nuts and seeds: eat raw, not roasted or tamaried, and without salt and sugar. Nut butters go well with fruit, toast, and celery sticks.

Oils: cold-pressed oils (it says so on the label) from health-food stores made from olive, flaxseed, canola, or sesame. Try to use organic whenever possible. Avoid margarines or unspecified sources of oils as well as cottonseed and palm oils.

Spices: salt and fresh herbs such as parsley, sweet basil, and oregano.

Sweeteners: you can use a small amount of maple syrup or rice syrup if you normally do not use these frequently in your diet.

Because it is difficult to eat on the elimination diet, I recommend approaching it this way. Pick two or three foods and eat them at one meal. Try to vary your foods as much as possible. The fewer foods you eat at a meal the easier it is to do. Don't skip meals. Eat frequently throughout the day, drink 2 glasses of water on rising and before bed, and lots of herbal tea or diluted fruit juice and water (1/3 juice to 2/3 water) during the day. Plan your meals one week ahead and ask lots of questions when you eat out.

What to Expect on Your Elimination Diet

Typically, you might feel worse than usual from the first through the fifth days. This can include fatigue, anxiety, headaches, irritability, or aggravations of your typical health problems. This is because your body can still be reacting to foods you ate last week (remember, this is based on intestinal-transit time), or you can be detoxifying the allergic foods. If these symptoms are severe, try taking 1000 mg of buffered vitamin C four times a day. If food allergies are contributing to your health problem, usually *by the fourth to sixth day you will start to feel free of your typical complaints and have increased well-being.*

You need to stay on this diet until your symptoms go away. Only in this manner can you know, when you start reintroducing foods, if the food you are testing is actually making your symptoms reappear. *If you still have symptoms, you cannot test a food.*

If you no longer have symptoms at the end of a week, you can start testing foods. If you still have symptoms at the end of the first week of the elimination diet, continue this restricted diet for several more days. Some people (not the majority) need fourteen or more days to clear out their systems.

If you've continued on the elimination diet and still suffer with health problems, then your health problems are probably not due to food allergies. Or you may be one of the rare folks who is allergic to the supposedly nonallergic foods you have been eating during the elimination diet. The elimination is based on *common* allergens. There are always exceptions. This is a potential drawback to this method.

Most skin tests are unreliable for identifying food allergies, and blood tests are very expensive and controversial. If you simply don't have the fortitude for an elimination diet, I recommend forking over the money for several different kinds of blood tests for food allergies, and going off the top ten to fifteen foods on each test or any foods that show up on two or more tests.

Reintroduction of Foods

Reintroduce one food a day.

To reintroduce and test a food, you need to have been symptom-free for two days. So, if you got rid of your symptoms on day seven, wait until day nine to test a food. Being symptom-free for two days confirms that you are really symptom-free.

Now you're ready to reintroduce the foods you eliminated from your diet. Try to use organic foods and test them in any order, even starting with your favorite ones first. If you have a reaction, you'll know it's that food. Do *not* start by testing foods you already know cause you trouble.

Eat the food in large amounts two meals in a row. For example, if you are testing corn, add corn tortillas, corn kernels, or popcorn, but do not add corn foods that contain a number of other ingredients. For example, don't add corn flakes that also contain other grains, nuts, and raisins. Add the food by itself.

Observe any "reactions" immediately after eating the food (now that you have unmasked or alerted your body, delayed reactions can become more immediate and easier to identify).

Observe how you feel all that day, night, and the next morning. If you have no reaction to that food, you may add it to your diet and continue testing other foods.

The exception is for people who have rheumatoid arthritis or any kind of severe joint pain. Those people need to reintroduce foods more slowly—*one food every two days.* This is because most reactions to reintroducing foods occur within 10 minutes to 12 hours, but joint pains may be delayed from 36 to 48 hours.

Related foods that need to be tested on separate days are: milk and cheese, egg whites and yolks, tap water and coffee or teas (without adding anything to them), food dyes (buy a set of food colorings, put a half teaspoon of each color in a glass of water, and test separately), and alcoholic beverages.

Introducing one food at a time simplifies matters by eliminating the confusion of reactions to various foods. If you react to all foods, you need a specialist well versed in natural approaches to food allergies.

What Might Be Your Food Reactions?

Reintroducing foods in this manner enables you to notice if you have any reactions, such as the return of your old symptoms, gastrointestinal upset, diarrhea, constipation, a sudden and severe bout of fatigue within two hours after eating, itching nose, phlegm in the throat, heart palpitations, redness of your ears, or an increase in allergic shiners (dark rings around and especially under the eyes).

Take note of your energy level, your mood (if you get depressed or weepy), how you sleep that night, how you feel waking up the next morning, and how your bowels move the next morning.

What to Do When You React to a Food

Stop eating all food, especially the one you just tested. If the reaction is mild, take 500 mg of buffered vitamin C, along with 250 mg of bromelain, every hour for three hours. Drink a lot of water. If the reaction stops and you are no longer reacting when you wake up the next morning, you can test a new food.

If your reaction continues, take the vitamin C and bromelain four to six times between meals, along with two pancreatic enzymes (do not take them if you have an ulcer), and add 2 Alka-Seltzer Gold in water two to three times that day, between meals. If you don't have that, put 1/5 teaspoon baking soda in 8 ounces of water and drink between meals two to three times that day, as needed. This regime decreases inflammation and allergic reaction. Don't add a food the next day. Wait till the third day.

When you wake up and feel clear, you are ready to test another food.

What to Do When You Find Your Food Allergies

When you find a "reactive" food, eliminate it from your diet for three months. During this time, consider an intestinal detoxification and rebuilding program (chapter 20) and assess your digestive enzymes (chapter 19). Supplement nutrients (see charts in chapter 20).

In the fourth month, reintroduce the suspected food. You do not need to do an elimination diet; just keep avoiding all your known allergy foods. You must be symptom-free before you add this food to be able to see if it creates reactions for you again. Add the food in the same manner you originally did. Watch for your reactions that day, night, and the next day.

If you don't have any reactions, this was probably not a true food allergy, but a secondary allergy caused by a toxic bowel, leaky gut, low nutrients, low digestive enzymes, etc. Now that you have healed these problems, you can handle this food. Add this food back into your diet two to three times a week, not every day. Be sensible and moderate.

If you react to this food again, strictly avoid this food for another six months. When your health is excellent, at some point down the road try this food one more time in the same manner described above. Sometimes a good long rest away from a food, as you are rebuilding your intestinal energy and your health reserves, will allow you to heal a food allergy.

If you reintroduce this food for a third time and you still react, you need to avoid this food permanently (three strikes and it's out). This food can now be labeled one of your *true food allergies,* meaning that eating this food truly stresses your body.

What to Do if You Seem to Be Allergic to Most Foods

I've seen frustrated patients who felt they had nothing left to eat. Blood tests, skin tests, and elimination diets had ruled out most normal foods. However, many of these people, after going through a bowel detoxification and rebuilding program, and/or supplementing their diets with digestive enzymes (low enzymes can cause delayed food allergies and poor absorption of nutrients), were able to eat more foods without problems. So don't suffer on long-term restrictive dietary regimes without trying to heal your intestinal tract. Consider:

- Bowel detoxification and rebuilding
- Digestive enzymes
- Other intestinal complications such as intestinal bacterial imbalance or parasites.

The Keys to Food Rotation

You may also consider rotating foods to cut down your reactivity. Food rotation is simply a way to avoid eating foods every day. You do this by eating a food every several days. For example:

Two-day rotation (mild problems): rice on Monday and Wednesday; corn on Thursday and Saturday.

Three-day rotation (moderate problems): rice on Monday and Thursday; corn on Friday and Tuesday.

Four-day rotation (severe problems): rice on Monday and Friday; corn on Saturday and Wednesday.

After three months, you should have fewer allergic reactions. If you still have problems, see doctors trained by the Academy of Environmental Medicine who use a technique called *provocative neutralization.* Call the American Academy of Environmental Medicine for doctor referrals in your area (913–642–6062).

TERRIBLE TWELVE-YEAR-OLD AND FOOD ALLERGIES

A twelve-year-old boy had many antisocial behaviors. He mutilated pets, lied, stole, damaged furniture, and had been having temper tantrums since he was one, as well as insomnia and a poor attention span. Dr. Theron Randolph, a pioneer in allergy medicine, discovered that the boy drank large quantities of orange juice and ate numerous hard-sugar candies daily. Dr. Randolph tested the boy and uncovered a number of food allergies. Strict avoidance of these foods as well as refined sugar normalized the boy's behavior, attitude, and schoolwork within a short period of time.

A CHIROPRACTOR'S "BAD" WRIST AND A CORN ALLERGY

Susan was a desperate chiropractor. Her wrists hurt so badly from chronic inflammation that she couldn't work. She reviewed her eating habits and noticed corn was a repetitive food in her diet. She loved corn and ate corn tortillas daily, as well as popcorn nightly. So she tried eliminating corn from her diet. Within one week her wrist problem disappeared. Upon reintroducing corn, it came back. Once she stayed off corn products, her wrist problem went away. By cleansing and rebuilding her intestinal tract over the next year, she was eventually able to eat corn products, moderately, without having a recurrence.

Supplements

Because you are allergic, you may have problems with supplements. Add one supplement a day. This allows you to identify any that may cause a problem. Remember, supplements are food. If taking all the supplements seems to not agree with you, try taking them throughout your meal. If that doesn't work, divide the dosage between two days, taking half of them one day and the other half the next. Avoid multiple vitamin/minerals (allergic people have difficulties handling these) for at least one to three months.

Three-Month Supplement Program to Heal Food Allergies

(Use all-hypoallergenic supplements and add one supplement a day.)

First Month, While Avoiding Suspected Foods

- *Vitamin C.* 1 gram twice a day (buffered form, corn-free is best).
- *Bioflavonoids.* 200 mg twice a day between meals.
- *Vitamin A.* 5000 IU once a day. (If you are pregnant, do not take vitamin A without doctor's supervision).
- *Pantothenic acid.* 500 mg one to three times a day.
- *Glutamine.* 500 mg to 1 gram two or three times a day.
- *Vitamin B complex.* 50 mg twice a day, along with 25 mg of B_6 (once or twice a day).
- *Flaxseed oil.* 3 capsules twice a day.
- *Lactobacillus mixtures.* 2 capsules twice a day.
- *Multiple mineral.* 1 twice day.
- *Digestive enzymes* with meals. Assess your need for these (chapter 19).
- Allergic cravings may sometimes be reduced with *chromium* (100 to 300 mcg) and *glutamine* (1000 mg two to three times a day) for several weeks.

Second Month. If your symptoms are better after one month, stop the between-meal supplements. Reduce all the other supplements that were taken three times a day to twice a day, and twice-a-day ones to once a day. If you are not a lot better at the end of the first month, then stay on the first-month program one more month. Check yourself against the list on pages 219–220 to see if you need to add specific nutrients.

Third Month. Take a multiple vitamin/mineral (if you can now tolerate these), B complex once a day, 1 to 2 grams of vitamin C a day, two essential oils twice a day, an antioxidant formula, and probiotics with dinner several times a week. See if you still maintain your improved health with this reduced dosage. If you don't, go back to the second-month dosage for another month. If you do well, you can stay on these maintenance dosages while you start to reintroduce some of your avoidance foods during the fourth month.

Dietary Suggestions to Help Heal Your Food Allergies

Eat fresh whole foods without additives, preservatives, sulfites, or pesticides, as much as possible.

Avoid eating heavily sprayed foods. Foods most likely to be heavily sprayed are peanuts, cottonseed oil, lettuce, citrus, apples, carrots, green and red bell peppers, any sugar-cane products, nonorganic spinach, and nonorganic dried fruits, such as raisins.

Eat foods that are high in essential oils and minerals, such as raw seeds, raw nuts, buckwheat, millet, legumes, and lots of berries, which are very high in flavonoids.

Nightshade Family: Potential Problems

In a small group of people, certain foods may cause toxic, though *not* allergic, reactions. An example is the nightshade family of foods: tomato, potato, eggplant, red pepper, and one nonfood item—tobacco. Nightshade sensitivities can aggravate and even cause arthritis for some people. If you have active symptoms of arthritis, you can test yourself in the same way you did the self-test for food allergies. These nightshade foods may cause other symptoms that have not been well described yet.

Dr. Jonathan Wright says, "A few of us are sensitive to nightshade foods, most are not. This underlines the old principle that nutrition is a highly individual matter."

Mind-Body Techniques

Reflex Points

Stimulate all digestive areas, thyroid, and pituitary gland. Also, wherever you have allergic reactions, stimulate that body part. (See reflexology charts at the end of chapter 20.)

Affirmation Exercise

Lie on your stomach and bend your knees. Raise the lower legs up in air. Cross your legs in the air one way as you inhale, and the other way as you exhale. Continue 25 times. When you are done, turn over. Lie on your back comfortably. Gently tap your breastbone ten times while saying, *"I heal my allergies. I heal my relationship with the outside world."*

Aerobic Exercise

Ten minutes to a half-hour a day of aerobic exercise is very helpful. The best exercise is the one you are motivated to do. Examples include walking briskly outside or on a treadmill, using a Stairmaster or rowing machine, swimming, etc. Just remember that you need to slightly alter what you do every six weeks to continue to positively stress your body to get results. If nothing else, at least vary the order of your exercises.

Mindfulness

Two-Part Exercise:

1. Sit quietly. In your mind's eye, travel through your mouth down the tube that is your intestinal tract. Imagine you can become a tiny little person, going inside yourself with a paintbrush. This paintbrush has a healing solution that can paint the lining of your intestinal tract with perfect health. Take your time and paint the entire length of your intestinal tract, from your mouth to your rectum. Focus longer on any part of your intestinal tract where you sense you have more trouble.

2. When you are done, sit quietly. Take a few gentle deep breaths. Remind yourself:

   "I am healing."

   "Food is my friend."

19 *Using Your Power Tools: Digestive Enzymes*

Estelle was sixty years old and so weak that in order for her to walk, her children had to hold her up under each arm. She suffered with fatigue, dizziness, and severe Raynaud's phenomenon, a spasm of the arterioles in the fingers and also, in Estelle's case, the tongue. It is aggravated by cigarette smoking, which Estelle had done heavily for years. Her doctors said there was no treatment for her condition.

Although Estelle had given up cigarettes, her condition had been worsening for two years. Her fingers and tongue were whitish blue and constantly tingled, and she had painful ulcers on some of her fingertips. Estelle had abdominal bloating most of the time, was frequently nauseated, and moved her bowels only once a week, which required much straining. Being understandably depressed, she had become unsocial and unkempt. She warned me, "I won't take handfuls of pills, mind you."

First, and most important, was to put Estelle on digestive enzymes. I also recommended several glasses of fresh fruit and vegetable juices daily. Knowing her attitude, that's all I recommended.

Two months later, Estelle showed up in my office groomed and smiling. She grabbed my hand and shook it like a strong truck driver. "I feel grand," she reported. "After two days my nausea left. After a week my bloating was gone. Now my hands don't tingle. But one thing . . ."

"What?" I asked.

"I don't look any younger." She winked and came at me like a bear, hugging me so hard my glasses fell off. Estelle's story shows how digestive tools can help illnesses that appear to have no treatment.

Digestive Enzymes in the Mouth

Digestion is an essential job the body performs, and digestive enzymes are the tools to do it right. Because food is inside the body for only a limited amount of time, these tools are needed to assist in breaking food down to optimize absorption.

Digestion is a cascade of events, sort of like a line of dominoes. One step occurs before another and each is essential for the rest to work correctly. Chewing food thoroughly is an important first step in the chain of digestive events.

As you chew, food mixes with saliva. Saliva contains starch-splitting enzymes that start the digestive process. Chewing also breaks food down into smaller particles, thus increasing the surface area of the food so the digestive tract can do a better job.

Remember, your stomach does not have teeth. The reason your mouth has teeth is so it can chew. This means that if you do not do an efficient job of chewing—if you eat too fast or are distracted by watching television, if you don't concentrate on thorough chewing—an undue burden is put on the rest of your digestive system. This may also mean that you don't need fancy supplements, diets, or formulas for your chronic bloating, abdominal discomfort, and coated tongue as much as you need more conscious and thorough chewing.

As food enters your mouth and is mixed with enzymes, this action notifies the rest of your digestion to get ready—food is coming. The same notification system takes place in your stomach. When food enters your stomach and stomach acid is released, this alerts other enzymes required farther down the digestive tract (secretin and pancreozymin in the duodenum and pancreatin from your pancreas) that they will soon be called into action.

Going back to our metaphor, if digestion were a series of dominoes, the thought, sight, taste, and chewing of food are the first dominoes. The release of gastric juice and hydrochloric acid is the next.

The Importance of Stomach Acid

There are cells lining the stomach that make gastric juice. Gastric juice contains a number of factors:

- *Intrinsic factors,* which help vitamin B_{12} absorption
- *Pepsin,* which helps digest protein
- *Hydrochloric acid (HCl)* (simply called stomach acid), which is essential for optimal digestion.

Stomach acid is so important because its helps activate the other digestive enzymes.

Hydrochloric acid helps digest protein. It does this by activating pepsin, which needs an acid environment to carry out its functions. Pepsin is a proteolytic enzyme, which means that it digests protein. This makes protein available to tissues throughout the body. Also, protein keeps vitamins and minerals bound into food particles. As pepsin breaks down protein structures in food, nutrients are liberated so they can be taken up by the blood stream and delivered to tissues.

Hydrochloric acid is needed in adequate amounts for most nutrients to get dissolved into the blood, especially calcium and iron.

Hydrochloric acid plays a protective role against unfriendly microorganisms, worms, and parasites. Food, water, and air are all potential routes for bacteria, fungi, and viruses to get into the body. These organisms are killed in the acid environment created by adequate secretion of stomach acid. In this way, stomach acid helps keep the stomach and small intestine sterile. Inadequate stomach acid contributes to an imbalance of intestinal flora.

The presence and overgrowth of unwanted organisms in the intestinal tract can inhibit nutrient absorption, burden the immune system, cause a "leaky gut," contribute to inflammation and ulcer formation, inhibit synthesis of vitamins (such as many of the B vitamins and vitamin K), as well as disrupt the balance of normally friendly organisms that perform essential functions in protecting us against diseases (see chapter 3).

Hydrochloric acid stimulates healthy digestion in the small intestine.

Adequate hydrochloric acid contributes to gallbladder, liver, and digestive health, and inadequate stomach acid may cause stress on these organs.

Low Stomach Acid

One commonly used medical textbook states that 10 to 15 percent of the general population doesn't make enough stomach acid. Over the past three decades, studies have shown that 10 percent of all retirees have inadequate levels of stomach acid and 5 percent make no stomach acid at all. These studies only tested initial levels of stomach acid and didn't account for stomach acid failures in the middle of meals. So the number of people with inadequate stomach acid levels is probably higher than generally realized. It is well known that as we age the rate of infection with a stomach bug called *H. pylori* increases, and this lowers the production of stomach acid, too.

Doctors are trained to think that if there is not enough acid in the stomach, the pancreas will simply take up the slack and finish the job. But what about the numerous essential actions stomach acid performs? The stomach requires an acid pH (acidity and alkalinity are measured in units called pH) of 1.5. The pH of blood is about 7.4. This means the body uses tremendous energy to make stomach acid one million times more concentrated than acid in the blood. The body must do this because stomach acid is so important!

What Causes Low Stomach Acid?

- Chronic stress.
- Poor eating habits.
- Nutrient deficiencies, especially a lack of zinc.
- Impaired immune-system functioning (immune system attacks the body, i.e., the stomach, instead of invaders).
- Oxidative damage (the body uses oxygen for many jobs, but in doing so can create damaging agents called free radicals).
- Aging.
- Variability in the amount of enzymes individuals require to function optimally and feel well.

Possible Signs of Low Stomach Acid

The Most Classic Signs of Low Stomach Acid

- Burping immediately after meals or up to one-half hour after a meal has ended.
- Abdominal bloating immediately after meals or up to one-half hour after eating.
- Food sitting uncomfortably in the stomach after eating.
- Loose stools in the morning.
- Painful dentures.
- Chronically coated tongue.
- Unexplained bouts of nausea.
- Using herbs but not improving from them.

Other possible symptoms of low stomach acid are: vague distress in the breastbone area immediately after eating, heartburn (can signal either too little or too much stomach acid), chronic diarrhea (especially in the morning), vomiting not related to a specific problem, and living healthfully but not feeling appropriately better.

Physical signs that may suggest low stomach acid are: dilated capillaries in the cheeks and/or nose not due to excessive alcohol consumption; general reddening of the facial skin, especially around the cheeks and forehead; medium to large acnelike pimples (rosacea) scattered around the nose and cheeks; areas of loss of pigment so the skin is blotched white (vitiligo); unusual pale skin coloring not due to illness or anemia; being prone to muscle cramps and spasms; nails that chip, break, or split and won't grow; taking nutritional supplements and getting worse; not responding to improvements in your diet or taking

Through the centuries, healers have recommended herbs from natural plants for numerous health conditions. But why is it that some people seem to get beneficial results from herbs, while other individuals do not? The answer may be stomach acid.

supplements; seeing undigested food in the stool; poor stress-coping skills; itching around your rectum; and chronic asthma, skin conditions, or anemias that do not respond to treatment.

It is important to remember that you may be low in stomach acid yet not have any symptoms. A commonly used medical textbook, *The Pharmacological Basis of Therapeutics,* says, "Indeed, some individuals who repeatedly fail to secrete hydrochloric acid may experience *no* gastrointestinal symptoms at all."

Stomach Acid and Herbs

One study has revealed that the primary active ingredients in herbs are usually low-molecular-weight compounds. These key healing factors are actually cleaved away from the other parts of the herbs by the action of stomach acid and pepsin. In this way, these vital compounds become available for transportation into the bloodstream. In this particular study, patients who responded favorably to herbs had more acid and pepsin in their stomach juices than patients who did not respond as favorably to herbs (*Planta Med* 1991;57:299–304).

How Do You Measure Your Stomach Acid?

Signs mentioned above.

Low minerals (ones that need to be solubilized—zinc, copper, and possibly chromium and calcium) on a hair-mineral analysis. Or, physical symptoms may suggest low stomach acid.

Microscopic stool tests evaluate the presence of undigested meat fibers. (See appendix B.)

The most accurate measurement of stomach acidity is the Heidelberg capsule test, a medical test to evaluate stomach acid. Without having been assessed by a Heidelberg test, you should not self-administer high dosages of stomach acid (above 30 grains), even though a "normal" stomach makes much more than 90 grains per meal. With this test, and working with an appropriate doctor, higher amounts can be used when proven to be necessary. The person being tested swallows a small pH-sensitive radio transmitter. Once inside the stomach, the transmitter records the acidity of the stomach. The person is given 2 teaspoons of baking soda in water (an alkaline solution) several times during the test. The transmitter radios to the receiver how effectively and quickly the stomach produces acid to reacidify the contents. This is called a stimulation challenge test and diagnoses stomach acid with a high degree of accuracy. This machine was invaluable in my practice for identifying acid problems in various patients.

Natural Remedies for Increasing Stomach Acid

To Increase Stomach Acid

Try one at a time for several days:
- *Lemon juice* sipped during meals.
- *Apple-cider vinegar.* 1 tablespoon mixed with 1 teaspoon of unprocessed honey, sipped during meals.
- *Vitamin B$_1$.* 100 mgs with each meal for a week, then reduce to once a day.
- *Stomach-glandular supplements.* 1 to 2 before each meal.
- *Extract of black pepper.* 5-mg capsule. This has been shown to enhance absorption of several nutrients.
- *Glutamine.* 200 to 500 mg two to three times a day is a normalizer for hydrochloric acid as well as bicarbonates farther down the intestinal tract.

If the above remedies do not help, you can try therapeutic trials of stomach-acid supplements with medical supervision. With therapeutic trials, the idea is to try taking stomach acid and see if your symptoms get better.

Stomach Acid Supplements

Begin with 1 500- to 650-mg *capsule* (not tablet) containing both hydrochloric acid (HCl) and 150 mg of pepsin. The pepsin helps the stomach acid work better. Start by taking one capsule after a few bites of food. *Do not take stomach acid on an empty stomach.*

If you have *no* discomfort (burning or warm sensations), add one capsule per meal. Often people with low stomach acid need an average of 10 to 30 grains per meal or 1 to 2 capsules with breakfast and 2 to 4 capsules with lunch and dinner.

If you experience pain, burning, or a strong warm sensation after taking the first trial stomach-acid capsules, drink milk, or take 1/4 teaspoon of baking soda in water or 1/2 cup of aloe vera juice mixed with an equal amount of water. *And stop taking the stomach acid!*

If you have trouble with betaine HCl, try glutamic HCl. Some sensitive individuals have problems with pepsin and need to take HCl without pepsin.

Take these capsules throughout your meal, mimicking the action of the stomach's natural secretions.

I often found that people required up to 30 grains in the beginning, but, over time, as they improved their health and diet, they could reduce this dose or even stop the stomach-acid supplements.

IMPORTANT: *Never take anti-inflammatory drugs (Indocin, Butazolidin, ibuprofin, aspirin, or cortisone) together with hydrochloric acid.* If you feel you are low in stomach acid but you regularly take any of these drugs, you must work with a doctor trained in hydrochloric acid supplementation.

If you need both stomach-acid and pancreatic-enzyme supplementation, take the stomach acid during meals and the pancreatic enzymes afterward.

STOMACH ACID HELPED RUTH'S IRON-DEFICIENCY ANEMIA

A doctor called me about a problem patient. Ruth had chronic anemia—iron-poor blood. But no matter how much iron the doctors gave her, she couldn't get better. Even iron shots helped only for a few days.

It turned out that Ruth was chronically constipated and burped frequently. Ruth lived far away from any office with a Heidelberg test. I advised the doctor to recommend that Ruth try stomach-acid supplements. Ruth started with one capsule per meal and ended by taking one at breakfast, two at lunch, and three at dinner. Her constipation went away in two weeks. In several months, her anemia cleared up and her energy climbed.

This is another case demonstrating that health is a complex web. All the iron in the world could not help Ruth—she needed to be able to *absorb* it.

Pancreatic Enzymes

Pancreatic enzymes help digest proteins, fats, carbohydrates and all fat-soluble vitamins (E, A, K, and D). They have an overall "surveillant" anti-inflammatory action in the body. Keep in mind that if your body does not make adequate pancreatic enzymes, you will not adequately digest many nutrients. Different people will develop different nutrient deficiencies, thus symptoms can vary widely. Comprehensive stool tests look under the microscope to make sure everything is digested, which is a good way to identify pancreatin enzyme deficiencies. (See appendix B for companies that do the stool tests.)

Symptoms of Low Pancreatic Enzymes and Malabsorption

- Gas, bloating, and indigestion one-half hour to several hours after eating meals (whereas low stomach acid usually causes problems *immediately* after eating).
- Chronic excessive intestinal gas.
- Chronic constipation, sometimes mild diarrhea, or alternating between the two.
- Frequent undigested food in stools.
- Frequent bubbles or grease in the toilet bowl around the stools.
- Floating or bubbling stools (because gas and grease float).

- Fat-soluble vitamin deficiencies (vitamins A, E, D, and K).
- Taking supplements or eating a good diet and not getting an appropriate improvement in health.

Pancreatic supplements

For low pancreatic enzymes, try taking 1 pancreatic enzyme supplement after each meal for three days. If you do not have adverse reactions, but your symptoms don't improve, increase the dosage to 2 after meals. In three days, if no changes occur, increase to 3 after meals. Standard doses are from several hundred to several thousand mg per meal. If you take pancreatic enzymes and your symptoms improve or go away, this is a good indicator that your body produced insufficient pancreatic enzymes for your optimal health.

Some very ill people require larger dosages, up to 6 pancreatic enzymes per meal—usually only for short periods of time—until they have a marked improvement in their symptoms. When you are taking high dosages of pancreatic enzymes, it is a good idea to rotate brands and types so you don't become allergic to any one source. People who need such a high dose of pancreatic enzymes usually have allergic tendencies.

WARNING: *Do not take pancreatic enzymes if you have ulcers or any kind of active inflammatory bowel condition.* There are no other known problems or contraindications for taking pancreatic supplements, except for being allergic to their sources. Most come from *pork* because pork enzymes are most similar to human enzymes. Others are from beef, lamb, and vegetarian sources. Enzymes from vegetable sources are said to work in a larger pH range and may help people who do not respond to enzymes from animal sources.

Some cases of pancreatic enzyme deficiencies are secondary to stomach-acid deficiencies. This is because the secretion of hydrochloric acid in the stomach is a stimulus to start pancreatic-enzyme release.

Working Out the Dosage

The dosage is trial and error, based on monitoring your symptom changes and overall sense of well-being. Pay close attention to your digestion, how many bowel movements you have, how rested you feel upon rising, how much energy you have throughout the day, and your original symptoms. Review signs of optimal digestion in chapter 1. The correct dose for digestive enzyme replacement is the one that optimizes your absorption, not just one that gets rid of overt symptoms, such as gas. The best thing to do is to pick two deficiency symptoms (see list on page 11) and monitor them to see if they improve.

Be patient. This is the self-exploration part of healing.

The problem is that "loud" symptoms, such as bloating and gas, are not perfect guides to use when adjusting your dosage. This is because the amount of enzyme that is needed to reduce your gas and bloating is not necessarily enough to reduce silent symptoms, such as poor absorption. You can ask your doctor to order a hair-mineral analysis every six months for a year to monitor your progress and watch the level of your minerals to evaluate absorption. Minerals to monitor are calcium, magnesium, copper, chromium, zinc, potassium, and selenium.

What Is Bile?

The liver makes bile and the gallbladder stores it. This is an essential part of digestion. Bile salts help digest fats, fat-soluble vitamins (A, E, D, and K), and essential oils. They also help to maintain normal intestinal microorganism balance, as well as overall digestive functioning.

Undigested fat can coat food and nutrients, which can cause poor absorption of iron and calcium. Thus, inadequate bile can put you at risk for bone loss, or osteoporosis.

Bile also carries waste products from the liver. This is an important component of detoxification. Detoxification keeps the body from building up levels of toxins and chemicals that put a burden on the immune system if not eliminated. In this indirect way, bile works with your immune system. Bile is alkaline. It neutralizes acid from the stomach and contributes to making the intestinal pH more optimal for digestion. Bile also helps you have optimal levels of friendly bacteria and gives your stools and urine much of their coloring.

Symptoms of Low Bile Salts

- Stools that are *persistently* pale brown, yellowish, or grayish (this does not mean singular events caused by dietary and lifestyle indiscretions).
- Discomfort, gas, bloating—especially after fatty meals.
- Heartburn.
- Vague and intermittent abdominal pains.
- Dull right-sided fullness several hours after eating.
- Chronic constipation.
- Fat-soluble vitamin deficiency signs. (See appendix C chart for these deficiency signs.)

You can find multiple digestive formulas with bile salts added. Take enough so that your stool is solid and a medium-brown color. If you don't take enough bile, your stool color won't change.

If you take too much, you can induce a mild to moderate greenish-tinged diarrhea with an unpleasant odor.

Bile salts come from animal sources, so allergic reactions are possible. Symptoms are: increased abdominal distress and allergic shiners (dark rings around the eyes), bouts of unexplained severe fatigue, red eyes, feeling worse, or continually burping up the tablet.

Never take bile salts for longer than two months. If your symptoms start to come back, you can go back on the bile salts for another two months, then stop again.

Note: If your stool is white or yellow for more than three days in a row, see a doctor immediately. A severe bile deficiency can herald serious health problems such as hepatitis, gallstones blocking bile ducts, pancreatic cancer, biliary cirrhosis, etc.

Some People Need Supplemental Enzymes and Others Don't

The reason is *biochemical individuality.* Roger Williams, Ph.D, D.Sc., was one of the fathers of nutritional medicine. He originated the concept of biochemical individuality in a book by the same name. He pointed out that the problem with standard medicine is that it is based on the classical textbook standards of physiology and anatomy (usually on the *male* body). William emphasized that different people, not textbook standards, often have very different needs.

In another of his books, *You Are Extraordinary,* Dr. Williams said that biochemical individuality is especially apparent in the realm of digestive enzymes. He explained that we all have tremendously different levels of enzymes. In a Mayo Clinic study of gastric juices from thousands of normal individuals, the hydrochloric acid contents varied over a 100- to 200-fold range! Williams said that the variation in the needs of individuals is not only astounding, it's also alarming. *Thus, even if you are in the normal range for digestive enzymes, that still may be too low for you to enjoy optimal health.*

20 *Detoxification and Rebuilding Programs*

The body is designed for housecleaning—ridding itself of many chemicals, drugs, and environmental pollutants, along with toxic substances that are inadvertently manufactured by the body itself in the daily process of metabolism. The better a body can rid itself of toxic substances, the better it can manage the other numerous activities involved in healthy living.

The reason it is important to discuss detoxification in a book about digestion is that to heal the digestive tract and digestive problems, it is sometimes helpful to do what is called a detoxification and rebuilding program. These programs assist your body in cleaning and healing the intestinal tract and supportive organs. These tools are especially helpful if you have not been getting results by improving lifestyle habits and taking natural supplements.

There are many varieties of detoxifying programs. Some are gentle, like the one recommended in this chapter, while some—such as lengthy detoxification programs offered by clinics—are more complex. Presented in this chapter is the program I recommended for many of my patients. I do not recommend embarking on detoxification programs or fasts without medical guidance.

Why Do We Need Detoxification Programs?

Modern medicine is miraculous in emergency situations, but in nonemergency situations, modern medicine rarely asks Why did this body get ill? How can we prevent it from getting ill again? How did this person's lifestyle contribute to this illness?

In contrast, *all* natural healing methods have one core philosophy in common: that *true healing starts from the inside out—not one part at a time.* Be it nutrition, osteopathy, cranial work, chiropractic, herbal medicine, naturopathic medicine, acupuncture, homeopathy, Chinese medicine, Ayurveda, reflexology,

Detoxification =

all the reactions necessary inside your body to help remove the buildup of waste materials, toxins, and unhealthy chemicals, and to promote better circulation, exchange of fluids and nutrients—all while not adversely stressing your health.

massage therapy, psychotherapy, or yoga—these schools of healing believe that the initial causes of illness must be removed and the body must be revitalized, cleansed, and become free of a number of possible *blockages* (nutritional, energetic, physical, emotional, structural, or breathing), *so that the body can be allowed to heal itself.*

The body has *innate wisdom* regarding its organs, tissues, and parts. When the body first gets out of balance, it still has this wisdom to be able to heal itself. This explains why the early stage of illness is the optimal time to attack a problem. If the problem goes on long enough, the healing aspect of the body (the wisdom) becomes distorted.

Everything in the body and mind is connected. A problem in the shoulder might be coming from the gallbladder. A stomach problem may be caused by poor dietary habits or by emotional upset. So a detoxification program also includes mind-body cleansing tools, such as affirmations or times of silence.

Detoxification, depending on the different healing disciplines, may be called by different names: healing leaky gut, identifying/eliminating allergies, identifying and treating malabsorption, clearing congestion, revitalization, restructuring, renutrifying, etc. All these terms refer to getting at the core of what is preventing the body from healing itself. Detoxification, or *cleansing,* as it is popularly referred to, means getting the body unblocked so it can call upon its natural resources to heal itself.

Reasons for a Detoxification Program

- Chronic digestive problems.
- Chronic health problems (occurring over three months, or recurring several times).
- Planning a pregnancy in the next several years and wanting to *prepare* your body. The health status of future moms and dads two years before conception influences the health of the yet-to-be-born baby. (Do not do a detox program within two to three months of getting pregnant.)
- Healing from an addiction. Work with a professional.
- Once-a-year house cleaning for prevention of disease.

In the future, techniques of detoxification will become more routine, like getting our teeth cleaned. This will be necessary because our water, air, and food are polluted. Our bodies have become chemical receptacles from external environmental contaminants. And consuming junk food creates internal pollution.

WARNING: People who should *NOT* do a detox program include: pregnant women; infants and children; those healing from *recent* surgery, chemotherapy, or radiation; and those experiencing active bowel disease, such as bleeding colitis, ulcers, or Crohn's disease.

The Body's Natural Detoxification System

Just as you need to clean your house on a regular basis to keep living in it comfortably, your body needs to "houseclean," or detox and rebuild, on a daily basis to be able to function optimally.

To attempt to meet the constant challenges of detoxification, the human body performs *biotransformation*. In this process, chemicals that are not easily dissolved or excreted from the body are transformed into new compounds that are more easily removed from the body.

To accomplish biotransformation, the body has three major tools:

1. Phase 1 and phase 2 enzymes, found in highest concentrations in the *liver* (the liver is the main player in the detoxification extravaganza).
2. Local repair stations found throughout the body.
3. Specific nutrients that support the functioning of the liver and the repair stations.

In order to help neutralize toxic intermediate compounds and/or enhance excretion of these compounds out of the body, an effective detoxification program uses a variety of antioxidants and associated nutrients, adequate protein and water in the diet, exercise or massage, as well as the avoidance of excessive sugar and refined carbohydrates.

It's common knowledge that exercise and water are essential to good health. However, most of us are not aware that one reason they are so important is that they are "mini tools" of detoxification. If used on a daily basis, they help our bodies detoxify, although to a lesser degree than embarking on a complete program.

Three Phases of Intestinal Detoxification and Rebuilding

1. Detoxification

The body has several routes of *elimination*—the skin, lungs, and intestinal tract (including the liver and gallbladder systems)—that assist in detoxification of the body.

Tools to enhance elimination through all these systems are part of a good detox program:

- Skin brushing.
- Walks in the open air (don't use sunscreen during this time).
- Deep breathing.
- Massage and exercise or hydrotherapy to increase circulation.
- Cleansing of the intestinal tract with fiber and bentonite drinks.
- Nutritional support through diet, herbs, and supplements.
- Enemas (colonics should be done only if working with a professional).
- Sweating.

2. Rebuilding

After detoxification, one must rebuild. Detoxifying without rebuilding creates a strain on the body that can actually be harmful. Rebuilding means eating carefully and avoiding stressor foods (see chapter 1 for details). This allows the inherent healing resources unleashed by the detoxification program to further heal. *Specific nutrients and foods help the liver detox, "reseed" friendly flora, and rebuild the intestinal lining.*

The rebuilding program should be three times as long as the detoxification program, because the body continues to cleanse and rebuild for some time after the initial detoxification phase. For example, after a one-week detox program, you should be on a rebuilding program for three weeks.

3. Maintenance

After the rebuilding program, it is time to establish optimal daily habits that include quality diet, exercise, and attitude.

JOHN, A RASH PHYSICAL TRAINER

John was an exercise trainer at a modern gym in the East Bay area of San Francisco. He had two secrets. First, he silently suffered with severe intestinal gas. Second, he had chronic itching from rashes.

When John wasn't cured by the usual medical sources, he came to see me. I explained that even though he ate well, undigested food and toxic metabolites were stressing his intestinal tract, and irritating his skin, causing rashes. John was instructed to do a home cleansing and rebuilding program and to take digestive enzymes with each meal. He was advised to eat a greater variety of fresh foods. John also learned how to rub certain reflex points on his feet to strengthen digestion and elimination. To reduce his stress, he was given relaxation and meditation tapes. In two months, John not only was free of gas and itching, but many other little complaints went away as well. From then on, John instructed his clients that digestion and elimination are just as important as exercise.

Tools for Detoxification and Rebuilding

Skin Brush

Skin brush the entire body in the morning and evening before a shower. I like brushes with a long handle for reaching the back. These can be purchased at your local health-food stores.

How to skin brush: Do 20 long strokes, moving from the extremities toward the torso (feet toward groin, hands toward armpits). Then brush in a crisscross pattern across the chest. Reach from the top of one shoulder, between the breasts (do not brush the breasts), down to the opposite side of the waist. Repeat this on the other side. Brush up to down. Then brush the abdomen in circles, going from right to left. Then the back, waist, and buttocks. Gently brush the face. Finish by brushing several times the major lymph areas (armpits and the upper inner thighs) toward the trunk of the body.

Deep Breathing and Visualization

Sit quietly and breathe in and out as slowly as you can, at least nine times, twice a day. At the end, inhale as much as you can and hold the breath. Visualize your body filled with "healing breath." On the exhale, visualize toxins leaving your body.

Other Tools

Daily, do at least 15 minutes of *exercise,* such as treadmill, exercise bike, or brisk walking. Exercise hard enough to break a sweat.

Go outside for at least 20 minutes a day. Get fresh air.

Do a cleansing *meditation* once a day (given at the end of this chapter).

If possible, get *hydrotherapy* from a naturopathic doctor, or, at the end of each shower, alternate hot and cold water 30 seconds each, increasing the circulation to the skin to enhance elimination.

Nutritional Support for Biotransformation

The following are foods to eat generously during detoxification, rebuilding, and maintenance.

Indoles to the Rescue. Indoles are substances in the *cabbage family* (Cruciferae)—broccoli, cabbage, Brussels sprouts, cauliflower, bok choy, green onions, and kale—that promote a detoxifying enzyme (glutathione s-transferase) in the lining of the intestinal tract and liver.

One study gave volunteers a drug while including Brussels sprouts and cabbage in their diet. Eating these vegetables stimulated a speedier metabolism and clearance of the drugs. According to the team that published this report in *Clinical Pharmacological Therapies,* Brussels sprouts and cabbage contain specific detoxifying indoles.

Bioflavonoids also stimulate this detoxifying enzyme. Fresh fruits, vegetables, soy, and milk thistle may all contribute in this way to healthy, gentle detoxification.

Eat adequate *protein* and generously add *onions* and *garlic* to your diet. Consume foods high in amino acids, such as *beans, nuts, fish, lean organic meats,* and *eggs.* Consume foods high in natural *antioxidants,* such as *red, yellow,* and *green vegetables, raw seeds, nuts,* and *fish.*

Season your food with *onions, garlic, rosemary, thyme, sage,* and *turmeric.* Add these seasonings at the end of cooking to preserve beneficial ingredients.

Avoid consumption of refined carbohydrates while on a detox program and for a moderate time afterward.

Consider supplementation with *glutathione.* This antioxidant helps remove toxic intermediate compounds and is therefore an important tool in healthy detoxification. Glutathione is made in the body from the amino acids cystiene and methionine. It is preserved by vitamin C. On the other hand, excessive use of alcohol and acetaminophen (Tylenol) rinse glutathione reserves out of the body.

There are many excellent commercial products for detoxification available through your local health-food stores and vitamin houses that can be used as the herbs for your detoxification program. Ask your health-food store attendant.

One-Week Detoxification Program

During this week, drink a high-fiber shake three times a day, one hour before meals. Keep eating solid meals three times a day—mostly fruits, vegetables, grains, seeds, nuts, and legumes. Eliminate stressor foods (see chapter 1). Eat organic foods and avoid animal products as much as possible. Do not fast and take these supplements. Do not fast without a doctor's supervision.

EASY FIBER SHAKE In a glass mix 2 teaspoons of psyllium husks (not seeds), 2 tablespoons of bentonite liquid (not powder), and diluted fruit juice (half water, half juice). Cover with a lid, shake for ten seconds, and drink immediately. This mixture gets thick very rapidly. Follow this with an 8-ounce glass of water to help the mixture go down.

All sources should be free of sugar, dairy, yeast, preservatives, salt, colorings, fructose, corn sweeteners, and low-caloric sweeteners. Do not use fiber sources with added herbs, such as cascara sagrada, senna, etc.

The *bentonite liquid* lines the intestinal tract so toxins that are released are not reabsorbed into the body. If you start to feel toxic, fatigued, or achy, try increasing the amount of bentonite liquid.

Daily Schedule for Mild One-Week Detoxification

Immediately on rising
Take 200 mg bioflavonoids, 1 gram of vitamin C, 2 green-powder capsules or one serving of a green powder source, 2 garlic capsules, plus a large glass of water. Skin brush and shower.

7:30 A.M.   High-fiber bentonite drink.

8:30 A.M.   Detox herbs. You have two choices: Take 3 to 5 capsules of one of the many commercial detoxifying formulas available at health-food stores, OR drink a detox tea: Slowly heat—do not boil—1/5 dropperful each of yellow dock, milk thistle, and burdock root in one cup of water.

9:00 A.M.   Breakfast
Fruit and whole-grain toast or cereal. 1 gram vitamin C, 1 B complex, 1 tablespoon of liquid minerals, 5,000 IU vitamin A, 2 pancreatic enzymes, 30 mg N-acetyl-cysteine, 3 probiotic capsules, and 50 mg glutathione.

10:00 A.M.   High-fiber bentonite drink.

11:30 A.M.   Detox herbs.

12:00 P.M.   Lunch
Big raw salad, or raw veggies, with grains or bread and/or beans or tofu. Take same nutrients as you had for breakfast, except do not repeat vitamin A.

2:30 P.M.   Detox herbs.

3:00 P.M.   High-fiber bentonite drink. Do afternoon exercise or breathing/affirmation program.

6:00 P.M.   Dinner
Steamed vegetables or stir-fry (use water, a little olive oil, and organic soy sauce), and/or whole grains and beans (example: whole-wheat noodles with black beans or tofu served over vegetables). Take same nutrients as at breakfast and lunch except do not repeat vitamin A, and add 2 oregano leaf and oil extract pills.

8:00 P.M.   Detox herbs.

Before bed: Take 2 garlic tablets, 2 blue-green algae or green-powder capsules, 200 mg of bromelain, and 2 antioxidants, plus a large glass of water.

The *detox herbs* cleanse the lining of the GI tract. The enzymes help to digest toxins and reduce inflammation. The combinations of all these items enhance the cleansing and elimination of the gastrointestinal tract. Do *NOT* take pancreatic enzymes if you have any kind of active ulcers or inflammatory bowel disease.

Three-Week Rebuilding Program

Eat well, avoid stressor foods, but add more protein foods (fish, chicken, or plant-based) back into your diet. Stop all detoxification supplements.

Add rebuilding nutrients.

- *Glutamine.* 1,000 mg three times a day.
- *Probiotics.* 2 capsules twice a day.
- *DGL.* 2 380-mg tablets, chewed 20 minutes before meals.
- *B complex.* twice a day.
- *Vitamin A.* 5,000 IU once a day.
- A *multiple vitamin/mineral*
- *Antioxidant.* 1 capsule twice a day.
- *Glutathione.* 50 mg, and *milk thistle,* 100 to 200 mg, one to two times a day.

When you finish with the rebuilding section, maintain yourself on a multiple vitamin/mineral and B complex and 1 antioxidant once a day.

Read chapter 1 again to learn about which protector foods to eat and which stressor foods to avoid. Now is the time to develop good eating and exercise habits, ones you will enjoy and maintain, and start living in a way that optimizes your life and does not drain you of energy.

While you are on any detoxification program, if at any time you begin to feel ill or worse than when you started:

1. Rest. Lie on your back with your feet elevated several feet above your heart.
2. Check the support lists to see if you've left important tools out of your program.
3. Do an enema with chamomile tea or filtered water.
4. Add another tablespoon of bentonite liquid to program.
5. If none of the above helps, stop the cleanse.

Mind-Body Techniques

Reflex Points

Sit quietly. Stimulate ALL the points on both feet, the heels, and up into the forelegs. Start with the intestine points, then the big toes, all the toes, the whole foot, the legs, and end with stimulating all the intestine points again. Stimulate deeply, search for sore spots, and work them out until they get less sore.

End the treatment with stroking movements from the foot upward into the groin. Use long, flowing movements. This stimulates the lymph glands to clear toxins. (See foot reflexology charts on pages 216–218.)

Two Exercises

1. Easy Twisting. Sit with arms overhead at a 45-degree angle. Take three deep breaths. Now inhale and twist to the left. Exhale and twist to the right. Repeat 25 times, gently. Inhale, exhale, then inhale deeply. Hold. Exhale and hold. Relax and lie down for several minutes.

2. Fire Breathing. Sit comfortably. Breathe deeply nine times. Now do rapid breathing from the lower abdomen. When you push your navel in, exhale out with an exaggerated force. This is called "fire breathing." Do this 25 times. At the end, inhale and hold your breath for 15 seconds. Exhale and hold the air out for 15 seconds. Sit quietly and relax. Do not do this if you have high blood pressure, are very weak, or get dizzy easily. Build up to doing this longer if you feel comfortable doing so.

Affirmation and Imagery

Lie down. Put on soothing music if you wish. Take three deep breaths. Tighten up your whole body, lifting your arms and legs and head up and tightening as hard as you can without hurting yourself. When you are as tight as you can get, suddenly let go. Let your whole body sink into the floor. Relax.

Pretend you have a flashlight in your mind's eye. The light is violet. Visualize going through your body, starting with your head, and shining this light into each corner and crevice of your body. See this light as sterilizing, cleansing, and rejuvenating your body. If you sense an area that needs extra attention, linger there as long as you feel is necessary. Try to use your intuition.

When you are done, affirm:

"I let go of toxins."
"I let go of obstacles."
"I cleanse."
"I heal."

Massage

Getting a massage at least once during the program is helpful, and daily would be fantastic. If you do so, drink several glasses of water after the massage.

Besides increasing your overall circulation and lymphatic drainage, touching stimulates varous healing points on the body. Massage with sesame oil is good for pulling out toxins.

Healing with Hydrotherapy

Sauna is excellent, for 20 minutes at a time. This is contraindicated if you have a serious illness, high blood pressure, or a neurological disease. End with a 30-second cold shower.

Place bay, eucalyptus, or ginger near the source of steam in order to inhale these cleansing herbs. This enhances detoxification. Herbal wraps and naturopathic hydrotherapy systems are excellent, too.

Programs of detoxification utilizing saunas, hydrotherapy, and colonics are available from Dr. Walter Crinnion at Healing Naturally. See appendix B.

Reflexology Zones for Digestion

1. Work out painful and gritty places until there is less pain and gritty sensation. Be gentle and use your breathing as well as the person's you are working on.

2. Grit: Lots of gritty points plus skin tags all over body (such as around neck and under arms) suggest tendency toward growing polyps in large colon. See a doctor.

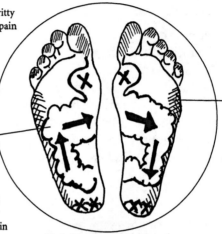

3. Finish with lymphatics: When intestinal massage is complete, stretch and rub lymphatics on tops and sides of feet toward upper leg and into thighs. Rub at least three times through in this direction.

Work from the right heel up the foot, across the instep to the left foot, and down to the left heel. This follows the path of the digestive tract.

Points down center of calf stimulate digestion, especially if points are sore or gritty.

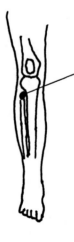

Stomach point (four fingers down from bottom of patella), which is a general digestive stimulatory point. Rub and hold for several minutes.

Reflex Points on the Feet

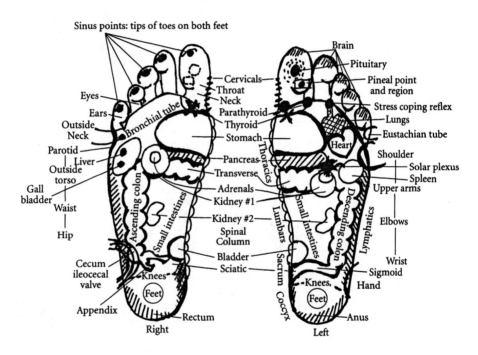

Sinus points: tips of toes on both feet

Brain
Pituitary
Pineal point and region
Stress coping reflex
Lungs
Eustachian tube
Shoulder
Solar plexus
Spleen
Upper arms
Elbows
Wrist
Sigmoid
Hand
Anus

Eyes
Ears
Outside Neck
Parotid
Outside torso
Gall bladder
Waist
Hip
Cecum ileocecal valve
Appendix

Cervicals
Throat
Neck
Parathyroid
Thyroid
Stomach
Pancreas
Transverse
Adrenals
Kidney #1
Kidney #2
Spinal Column
Bladder
Sciatic
Rectum

Liver
Bronchial tube
Ascending colon
Small intestines
Knees
Feet

Heart
Thoracics
Lumbars
Sacrum
Coccyx
Small intestines
Descending colon
Lymphatics
Knees
Feet

Right

Left

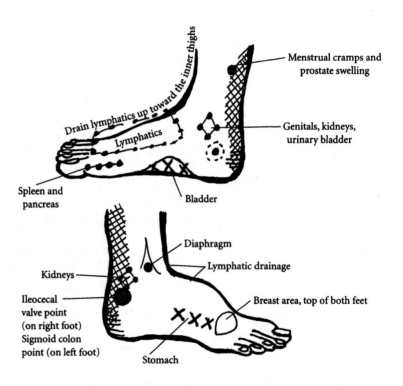

Drain lymphatics up toward the inner thighs

Lymphatics

Menstrual cramps and prostate swelling

Genitals, kidneys, urinary bladder

Spleen and pancreas

Bladder

Kidneys

Ileocecal valve point (on right foot) Sigmoid colon point (on left foot)

Diaphragm

Lymphatic drainage

Breast area, top of both feet

Stomach

Easy-Glance List of Symptoms Suggesting Inadequate Levels of Nutrients

Vitamin A
- History of Crohn's disease or ulcerative colitis
- Peptic ulcer, poor night vision, takes exceptionally long to see once you walk into a dark room (dark adaptation), dry eyes, acne or history of chronic acne, tendency toward recurrent infections (such as lung or urinary tract), tendency toward food allergies and/or diarrhea, rough "chicken-skin" on arms or thighs, frequent colds and flu during winter months.

Vitamin C
- Slow intestinal transit time, bruises easily, puffy gums, gets ill easily, chronic joint and/or soft tissue problems.

Vitamin B6
- Poor dream recall, excess ear wax, premenstrual syndrome, water retention, swollen, stiff fingers in the early morning (making it hard to bend fingers into the palm of the hand), carpal tunnel syndrome, and a number of the signs of inadequate levels of magnesium.

Vitamin B5
- Tendency toward gas and/or constipation, burning or cramping feet and legs, insomnia, fatigue (especially on rising and after exercise).

Vitamin B Complex
- Slow intestinal transit time, fatigue (especially in the afternoon), mood swings, sores/cracks on tongue or mouth, signs of inadequate levels of magnesium and/or essential fatty acids.

Magnesium
- Tendency toward constipation or irritable bowel syndrome, muscle spasms/cramps/twitching, irritability, noise sensitivity, excess ear wax, premenstrual syndrome, irregular heartbeat, depression and a sense of "doom," signs of inadequate levels of B_6 and essential fatty acids.

Essential Fatty Acids
- Tendency toward constipation and secondary hemorrhoids or fissures, inflammatory soft tissue or joint problems, rough "chicken-skin" on upper arms and

thighs, dandruff, dry brittle hair, ridged, cracking nails, dry skin, cracks in the heels and between fingers and toes, chronic respiratory problems, and chronic pain.

Chromium
- Blood sugar problems (high and low), Syndrome X, afternoon energy slump, fatigue, shakiness, mood swings.

Calcium
- Muscle cramps, nervousness, irregular heartbeat, headaches, low bone density or frequent fractures.

Zinc
- Tendency toward chronic or recurrent diarrhea, Crohn's disease, peptic ulcers, infections, white spots on fingernails, poor and/or slow wound healing, acne, rashes, can scar easily.

Amino Acid Imbalance
- Poor resistance and/or healing, mood swings, attention deficit hyperactivity disorder, poor response to a variety of treatment protocols for various health problems.

Specific Problems

Thyroid:
- Sluggish digestion and/or constipation
- Food "sits in stomach"
- Slow intestinal transit time
- Bloats easily, frequently feels cold, has multiple food allergies, weight gain, slow reflexes, low voice, mood swings, yellowish tone to skin or palms of hands not due to diet, and attention deficit hyperactivity disorder.

Cystic Breasts:
- Excess caffeine consumption, inadequate levels of vitamins E, D, B, and iodine and calcium.

Hemorrhoids:
- Inadequate levels of bioflavonoids, vitamins E and A, and essential fatty acids.

Chronic Headaches:
- Inadequate levels of any of the following: magnesium, calcium, vitamin B_1, and PABA.

Inadequate Stomach Acid:
- Signs of indigestion like burping, gas, and bloating immediately after a meal.

Inadequate Pancreatic Enzymes:
- Signs of indigestion such as gas and bloating from an hour and a half to many hours after eating a meal.

Resources

DIETARY SUPPLEMENTS

A wide number of companies formulate numerous dietary supplements that may be nutritionally supportive for specific digestive disorders. For your convenience, some are listed below, along with phone numbers for ordering. Naming these products does not constitute any endorsement of one product over any other.

If you are working with a licensed professional, they can order these products.

Gas and Bloat

Inflazyme Forte. American Biologic 800-227-4473
Beano. AkPharma Inc. 888-773-5433
Gentian-Angelica Bitters Compound. Eclectic Institute Inc. 800-332-4372
Muco-plex. Enzymatic Therapies 800-558-7372
Herbal Digestant. Natural Choice 801-479-8610
Say Yes To Beans. Nature's Plus 800-645-9500
Jarrow-Zyme Plus. Jarrow 310-204-6936, 800-726-0886
Digest Herbal. Zand 800-800-0405

Numerous companies make digestive enzyme formulas and beneficial bacteria products.

Heartburn

Gastro Smooth and Peppermint Plus. Enzymatic Therapies 800-558-7372
Quiet Harmony. Health Concern 800-233-9355
Digest Enzymes. Natural Choice 801-479-8610
Sano-Gastril. NutriCology 800-545-9960
Stomach Chi. OHCO 303-647-2466
Prelief. 888-773-5433
Acid Ease. Prevail 800-248-0885
Liquid Calcium/Magnesium (buffered). N.F. Formula 800-547-4891

Aloe Products, papaya enzymes, and beneficial bacteria may also be helpful.

Constipation

Garli-Phyll. Jarrow 310-204-6936, 800-726-0886
Simone Protective Pharmaceuticals #6, 609-896-2646

Cleansing Fiber and *Cleansing Laxative.* Zand 800-800-0405
Cascara Plus. N.F. Formula 800-547-4891

Many companies offer high fiber and herbal products.

Diarrhea

Gastro-Smooth. Enzymatic Therapies 800-558-7372
Inner Ecology's Acidophilus. Prevail 800-248-0885
GastroCleanse. NutriCology 800-545-9960
The Ultimate Florazyme. 800-843-6325
Beneficial Bacteria Products. Natren 805-371-4737, 800-992-3323
Stomach Chi. OHCO 303-647-2466
Chloro-Combo (contains allantoin). World Organics 714-893-0017

Many companies offer beneficial bacteria products.

Diverticular Disorders

Bastyr Formula B. Eclectic Institute Inc. 800-332-4372
Sialex. Ecological Formula 800-888-4585
The Ultimate FloraZyme. The Ultimate Life Co. 800-843-6325

Many companies make fiber, aloe, bromelain, and beneficial bacteria formulas, all of which may offer nutritional support for this condition.

Hemorrhoids

Myodern topical cream. N.F. Formula 800-547-4891

Many companies sell fiber, bioflavonoid, aloe vera, and essential oil (flax, borage, evening primrose oil, etc.) products, which may all be helpful for this condition.

Examples of fiber sources, most of which can be obtained from local health-food stores or direct houses are: Yerba Prima, Jarrow, Zand, Aloe Life Fiber Mate, Twin Labs, Soloray, and Simone Protective Pharmaceuticals #6

Inflammatory Bowel Disorders

Bastyr Formula B. Eclectic Institute Inc. 800-332-4372
 Sialex and *Colixen.* Ecological Formula 800-888-4585
RF Plus. N.F. Formula 800-547-4891

Oxygenators may be helpful, such as:
Dioxychlor. American Biologic 800-227-4473
Aerobic 07. Aerobic Life 800-798-0707
Oxy Caps and/or *Oxy-Cleanse.* Matrix Health Products 800-736-5609
Chloro-Combo (contains allantoin). World Organics 714-893-0017

Ulcers

Gasta-Comp. Bio-Design 888-577-4888

Bastyr Formula B. Eclectic Institute Inc. 800-332-4372
Helicobactrin. Ecological Formula 800-888-4585
DGL and *Gastro-Smooth.* Enzymatic Therapy 800-558-7372
DGL Plus. Nu Biologic 800-332-3130
RF Plus with Bismuth. N.F. Formula 800-547-4891
Sano-Gastril and *Gastro Cort II.* NutriCology 800-545-9960
DGL Plus. Progressive Laboratories/Kordial Products 800-527-9512
DGL. Priority One 800-443-2039

There are a wide variety of aloe products that may be helpful.

Tourist's Revenge (*Turista*) and 24-Hour Intestinal Flu

Bastyr Formula B. Eclectic Institute Inc. 800-332-4372
Gastro-Smooth. Enzymatic Therapy 800-558-7372
Garli-Phyll. Jarrow 310-204-6936, 800-726-0886
EHB herbal product. N.F. Formula 800-547-4891
GastroCleanse. NutriCology 800-545-9960
Stomach Chi. OHCO 303-647-2466

Irritable Bowel Syndrome (IBS)

Anti-Spaz. Crystal Star 209-532-4449
Sialex and *Colixen.* Ecological Formula 800-888-4585
Gastro-Smooth +/o Peppermint+. Enzymatic Therapy 800-558-7372
RF Plus. N.F. Formula 800-547-4891
Valerian Blend. Soloray 801-626-4956
Mynax. Koehler 206-424-6025
Sialex. Cardiovascular Research 800-351-9429

Detoxification Programs (several days to one week)

Arise and Shine. Arise & Shine Herbal Products 800-688-2444
AM/PM Ultimate Cleanse. Nature's Secret 800-29-SECRET
PhytoPro. *N.F. Formula 800-547-4891
GastroCleanse. NutriCology 800-545-9960
Sonnes No. 6 and No. 9 800-544-8147
Quick Cleanse Kit. Zand 800-800-0405

Parasites

Wormwood Combination. Kroeger Herb 800-225-8787
Phytofuge. *N.F. Formula 800-547-4891
Artimisia. NutriCology 800-545-9960
Citrus-seed Extract (available in 3 strengths) and *Tricycline.* NutriCology 800-545-9960
Paradex. *Nu Biologic 800-332-3130
ParaGard. *Tyler 503-661-5401, 800-869-9705
Awareness Products 800-265-9475

Candida-Related Complex

Aqua Flora. Made by East West and distributed by health-food stores and Women's International Pharmacy 800-279-5708

Candimycin and *ParaBan.* Enzymatic Therapy 800-558-7372

Phytostan. *N.F. Formula 800-547-4891

Citrus-Seed Extract (available in three strengths, including *Paramycocidin Forte*) and *Tricycline.* NutriCology 800-545-9960

Candida Albicans. *Priority One 800-443-2039

Kolorex. Infinity Health 800-733-9293

Colic

Chamomile Catnip Formula. Eclectic Institute 800-332-4372

Beneficial bacteria formulas are offered by many companies and may be helpful for both mother and child.

Hypoallergenic Protein Sources

Secure Proper Nutrition, Inc., offers a predigested white fish protein powder for people who are allergic to common sources of protein, 800-555-8868. This product also promotes enhanced digestion.

Green Products

Green Magma. Green Foods Corp. 800-222-3374

Blue Green Algae. Klamath 800-327-1956

ProGreens. NutriCology 800-545-9960

Many companies carry quality "green food products." Just make sure sources are free of heavy metals or other contaminants.

Water

Micro Water is available through High Tech H2O. Contact Bill Johnson, 510-820-8829. They have water filters that alkalinize and oxygenate water.

The Good Water Company, Inc., of Santa Fe, New Mexico, 800-471-9036, creates customized water systems throughout the United States. This company installs reverse osmosis water filters in the home. They can then reintroduce minerals into the filtered water. These minerals can be formulated from a personal physician's recommendation.

Referrals for Holistic Professionals

Call these organizations for referrals in your area:

American Academy of Environmental Medicine 913-642-6062

American Association of Acupuncture and Oriental Medicine 919-787-5181

American Association of Naturopathic Physicians 206-323-7610

American Botanical Council (for herbalists) 512-331-8868

American Chiropractic Association 703-276-8800
American College for Advancement in Medicine 800-532-3688
American Holistic Medical Association 919-787-5181
Dr. Rapp's Practical Allergy Research Foundation 800-787-8750
International and American Association of Clinical Nutritionists 972-250-2829

Specialists in Nutritional/Digestive Evaluation

Dr. Randy Baker, *The Pacific Center for Integral Health.* 408-476-1886

Dr. Walter Crinnion, *Healing Naturally,* offers in-depth digestive and nutritional evalua-
tions, thermal chamber chemical detoxification, along with hydro and colonic
therapies. 425-821-8118

Dr. Stephen Feig specializes in digestive problems and parasitology. 201-376-8353

The *Tahoma Clinic* in Kent, Washington, has a staff of doctors trained in all aspects of
digestive evaluation and health. This clinic has numerous resources. Next door is a
health-food store with a complete health book section that sells through mail-
order. 206-854-4900.

Dr. Barry Taylor, *New England Family Health Care Center*, has taught intestinal detoxification around the country (Love Your Body seminars) and is an expert in nutritional support for digestive health. 617-254-7700

Direct Order

These companies carry many different nutritional lines and offer many of the
products mentioned earlier. They mail directly to your home, send a catalog
upon request, and offer assistance.

Emerson Ecologies Inc. 800-654-4432
Health by Us 800-784-5567
Key Pharmacy 206-878-3900
Kroeger Herbs 303-837-8544
Swansons 800-437-4148
The Vitamin Trader 800-334-9310
Wellness Health & Pharmacy 800-227-2627
Women's International Pharmacy 800-279-5708

Laboratories

There are a number of laboratories that perform various types of nutritionally
related assessments. Your doctor may not be familiar with these laboratories or
tests. Once you inform your doctor, he or she can call for catalog of tests as well
as assistance in interpretation of results.

Digestive Stool Evaluation and Parasite Testing

Chelsea Biologics prefers to do testing on premises in New York City, but has kits available as well. Written up in *POZ* magazine, dedicated to latest information on AIDS,
as the most comprehensive lab for parasite testing. 212-242-2081

Diagnos-Techs, Inc. 206-251-0596

Great Smokies Diagnostic Laboratory 704-253-0621, 800-522-4762
Immuno-Sciences Lab, Inc. 310-287-1884, 800-950-4686
Institute of Parasitic Diseases 602-955-4211
Jetti Katz Infectious & Tropical Disease Lab (free consultations—if you are using this lab—available between your doctor and a board certified physician in infectious and tropical diseases at this lab about your case). 212-472-3542, 877-472-3540
Meridian Valley Clinical Laboratory 206-859-8700, 800-234-6825

Mineral Analysis and Other Nutritional Tests

Doctors' Data Inc. & Reference Laboratory also performs a Diet Analysis. 603-231-3649, 800-323-2784
Meridian Valley Clinical Laboratory 206-859-8700, 800-234-6825
Monroe Medical Research Laboratory, Inc. 914-351-5134
SpectraCell Laboratories, Inc. 713-621-3101, 800-227-5227

Intestinal Permeability Test (Leaky Gut)

Diagnos-Techs, Inc. 206-251-0596, 800-878-3787
Great Smokies Diagnostic Laboratory 704-253-0621, 800-522-4762
Meta Metrix Medical Laboratory 800-221-4640

Stomach Acid Test (Heidelberg Gastric Analysis)

Meridian Valley Clinical Laboratory 206-859-8700, 800-234-6825

Ulcer-bug Test (*H. pylori*)

Great Smokies Diagnostic Laboratory 704-253-0621, 800-522-4762
Immuno Laboratories, Inc. 305-486-4500, 800-950-4686
(Most laboratories test for this now.)

Newsletter

Nutrition & Healing 800-528-0559

APPENDIX C

References

INTRODUCTION

Jackson, A. "Reflexology Improves Sense of Well-Being." *Nursing Times* 92(51):50 1996.

Jackson, A. "Reflexology Relieves Migraines." *Nursing Times* 92(44):57 1996.

Trousdell, P. "Reflexology Meets Emotional Needs." *Journal of the Association of Complementary Medicine* 1996; 14 (11): 9–12.

CHAPTER 1. UNDERSTANDING YOUR DIGESTION

American Journal of Digestive Diseases. "Passage of Native Proteins Through the Normal Gastro-Intestinal Wall." Editorial in *American Journal of Digestive Diseases* 1935; 2:324–325.

Bray, George W. "The Hypochlorhydria of Asthma in Childhood." *Quarterly Journal of Medicine* (January 1931):181.

Challa, Anjana, et al. "Interactive Suppression of Aberrant Crypt Foci Induced by Azoxymethane in Rat Colon by Phytic Acid and Green Tea." *Carcinogenesis* 1997; 18(10): 2023–2026.

Drossman, D. A., et al. "Bowel Patterns Among Subjects Not Seeking Health Care." *Gastroenterology* 1982; 83:529–534.

Dvorak, Ann M. "Vitamin A in Crohn's Disease." Letter to *The Lancet* (June 14, 1980): 1303–1304.

Evans, Mary Ann, M.D. and Eva P. Shronts. "Intestinal Fuels: Glutamine, Short-Chain Fatty Acids, and Dietary Fiber." *Journal of the American Dietetic Association* 1992; 92: 1230–1246.

Fromm, David, M.D. "Gastric Mucosal 'Barrier.'" *Gastroenterology* 1979; 77(2).

Harvey, R. F., S. Y. Salih, and A. E. Read. "Organic and Functional Disorders in 2000 Gastroenterology Outpatients." *The Lancet* (March 19, 1983): 632–634.

Van Der Hulst R.R.W.J., M.D., et al. "Glutamine and Intestinal Immune Cells in Humans." *Journal of Parenteral and Enteral Nutrition* 1997; 21:310–315.

Walker, W. A., M.D., and K. J. Isselbacher, M.D. "Intestinal Antibodies." *New England Journal of Medicine* 1977; 297(4): 767–773.

Wilmore, Douglas W., M.D. "Metabolic Support of the Gastrointestinal Tract." *Cancer* 1997; 79:1794–803.

Wright, Jonathan V., M.D. *Dr. Wright's Book of Nutritional Therapy: Real-Life Lessons in Medicine without Drugs.* Emmaus, PA: Rodale Press, 1979.

Wright, Jonathan V., M.D. *Dr. Wright's Guide to Healing with Nutrition.* Emmaus, PA: Rodale Press, 1984.

CHAPTER 2. FIBER AND WATER

Bland, Jeffrey, ed. *Medical Applications of Clinical Nutrition.* New Canaan, CT: Keats Publishing, 1983.

Burkitt, Denis P., M.D. "Dietary Fiber: Is It Really Helpful?" *Geriatrics* 1982; 37(1):119–126.

Connell, Alastair M., M.D. "Natural Fiber and Bowel Dysfunction." *American Journal of Clinical Nutrition* 1976; 29:1427–1431.

Eades, Michael R., M.D. and Mary Dan Eades, M.D. *Protein Power.* New York: Bantam, 1996.

Fiore, P., et al. "Possible Side Effects on Vitamin A Stated Due to Fiber Supplementation in Diabetic Children." Letter to the Editor. *Nutrition* 15 (2):1999.

FDA Total Diet Survey 1982–1986 and FDA Pesticide Program Residue Monitoring 1992, 1993.

Harvey, R. F., E. W. Pomare, and K. W. Heaton. "Effects of Increased Dietary Fibre on Intestinal Transit." *The Lancet* (June 9, 1973):1278–1280.

Jacobs, Lucien R. "Effects of Dietary Fiber on Mucosal Growth and Cell Proliferation in the Small Intestine of the Rat: A Comparison of Oat Bran, Pectin, and Guar with Total Fiber Deprivation." *American Journal of Clinical Nutrition* 1983; 37: 954–960.

Sears, Barry. *Enter the Zone.* New York: Regan Books, 1995.

Williams, Roger J. *Physicians' Handbook of Nutritional Science.* Springfield, IL: Charles C. Thomas, 1975.

Williams, Roger J., ed., and Dwight K. Kalita, ed. *A Physician's Handbook on Orthomolecular Medicine.* New York: Pergamon Press, 1977; New Canaan, CT: Keats Publishing, 1979.

UC Berkeley Wellness Letter. "Water Works." *UC Berkeley Wellness Letter* September 1998; 14(12):2.

CHAPTER 3. INTESTINAL PROTECTORS

Anderson J. W. "Effect of Fermented Milk (Yogurt) Containing L. Acidophilus L1 on Serum Cholesterol in Hypercholesterolemic Humans." *Journal of the American College of Nutrition* 18 (1):43–50 (1999).

Cummings J. H. and G. T. MacFarlane. "Role of Intestinal Bacteria in Nutrient Metabolism." *Journal of Parenteral and Enteral Nutrition* 1997; 21(6):357–364.

Gorbach, Serwood L., M.D. "Efficacy of *Lactobacillus* in Treatment of Acute Diarrhea." *Nutrition Today* Supplement 1996; 31(6):19S–23S.

Grönlund, Minna-Maija, et al. "Fecal Microflora in Healthy Infants Born by Different Methods of Delivery: Permanent Changes in Intestinal Flora after Cesarean Delivery." *Journal of Pediatric Gastroenterology and Nutrition* 1999; 28:19–25.

Majamaa, Heli, M.D. and Erika Isolauri, M.D. "Probiotics: A Novel Approach in the Management of Food Allergy." *Journal of Allergy and Clinical Immunology* 1997; 99:179–85.

Oberhelman, Richard A., M.D., et al. "A Placebo-Controlled Trial of *Lactobacillus* GG to Prevent Diarrhea in Undernourished Peruvian Children." *Journal of Pediatrics* 1999; 134: 15–20.

Senecca, H. "Bacterial Properties of Yogurt." *American Practitioner Digestive Treatments* 1950; 1:1252–1259.

Shahani, K. M. and A. D. Ayebo. "Role of Dietary Lactobacilli in Gastrointestinal Microecology." *American Journal of Clinical Nutrition* 1980; 33: 2448–2457.

Walker, W. Allan and Linda C. Duffy. "Diet and Bacterial Colonization: Role of Probiotics and Prebiotics." *Journal of Nutritional Biochemistry* 1998; 9:668–675.

Young, R. J., et al. "Therapeutic Efficacy of *Lactobacillus Plantarum* 299V in Chronic Recurrent Abdominal Pain of Childhood." *Journal of Pediatric Gastroenterology and Nutrition* 1997; 25(4):465.

CHAPTER 4. USING YOUR MIND-BODY LINK TO MAXIMIZE DIGESTIVE WELLNESS

Achterberg, Jeanne. "Mind and Medicine: The Role of Imagery in Healing." *Journal of the American Society for Psychical Research* 1989; 83(2):93–100.

Addolorato, Giovanni, M.D., et al. "Anxiety and Depression: A Common Feature of Health Care Seeking Patients with Irritable Bowel Syndrome and Food Allergy." *Hepato-Gastroenterology* 1998; 45:1559–1564.

Braud, W. "Distant Mental Influence of Rate of Hemolysis of Human Red Blood Cells." *Journal of the American Society for Psychiatric Research* 1990; 84(1):1–24.

Benson, Herbert. *The Relaxation Response.* New York: Avon Books, 1975.

Benson, Herbert. *Beyond the Relaxation Response.* New York: Berkeley Books, 1984.

Benson, Herbert. *Timeless Healing.* New York: Fireside, 1997.

Brigham, D. D. and P. O. Toal. "The Use of Imagery in a Multimodal Psychoneuroimmunology Program for Cancer and Other Chronic Diseases." Chapter in *Mental Imagery,* Robert G. Kunzendorf, ed. New York: Plenum Press, 1991.

Byrd, R.C. "Positive Effects of Intercessory Prayer in a Coronary Care Unit Population." *Southern Medical Journal* 1997; 8:7.

Collins, S. M. "Is the Irritable Gut an Inflamed Gut?" *Scandinavian Journal of Gastroenterology* 1992; Suppl.192:102–105.

Dossey, L. *Healing Words: The Power of Prayer and the Practice of Medicine.* New York: HarperCollins, 1997.

Miller, R. N. "Study on the Effectiveness of Remote Mental Healing." *Medical Hypotheses* 1982; 8: 481–490.

Rein, G. "A Psychokinetic Effect on Neurotransmitter Metabolism." *Research in Parapsychology,* 1995. Metuchen, N.J.: Scarecrow Press, 27–80.

Rider, M. S. and J. Achterberg. "Effect of Music-Assisted Imagery on Neutrophils and Lymphocytes." *Biofeedback & Self Regulation* 1989; 14(3): 247–257.

Rider, Mark S., et al. "Effect of Immune System Imagery on Secretory IgA." *Biofeeedback & Self Regulation* 1990; 15(4):317–333.

Schlitz, M. "Intentionality and Intuition and Their Clinical Implications: A Challenge for Science and Medicine." *Advances: the Journal of Mind-Body Health,* 12(2):819.

Simonton, O. C., S. Matthews-Simonton, and J. Creighton. *Getting Well Again.* Los Angeles: Tarcher, 1978.

Smith, C. W., et al. *Imagery and Neutrophil Function Studies: A Preliminary Report.* Unpublished manuscript, Michigan State University, 1983.

Tusek, Diane L., et al. "Guided Imagery: A Significant Advance in the Care of Patients Undergoing Elective Colorectal Surgery." *Diseases of Colon and Rectum* 1997; 40:172–178.

Uehara A., et al. Gastric Antisecretory and Antiulcer Actions of Interleukin-1. "Evidence of the Presence of an 'Immune-Brain-Gut' Axis." *Journal of Clinical Gastroenterology* 1992; 14 Suppl:S149–55.

Weidermann, C. J., et al. "Vasoactive Intestinal Peptide Receptors in Rat Spleen and Brain: A Shared Communication Network." *Peptides* 1988; 9: 21–8.

Whitcomb, David C., M.D. and Ian L. Taylor, M.D. "A New Twist in the Brain-Gut Axis." *American Journal of Medical Science* 1992; 304(5):334–338.

Whorwell, P. J., L. A. Houghton, E. E. Tayor, and D. G. Maxton. "Physiological Effects of Emotion: Assessment via Hypnosis." Comment in *The Lancet* (August 1992):434.

CHAPTER 5. EASY WAYS TO GET RID OF GAS AND BLOATING

Ferguson, Anne and Stephan Strobel. "Immunology and Physiology of Digestion." In *Clinical Reactions to Food,* edited by M. J. Lessof. New York: John Wiley & Sons, 1983.

Levitt, Michael D., M.D. "Role of Gas in Functional Abdominal Pain." *Southern Medical Journal* 1984; 77(8):962–964.

Levitt, Michael D., M.D., et al. "Studies of a Flatulent Patient." *New England Journal of Medicine* (July 1976):260–262.

New England Journal of Medicine. "Intestinal Gas Production—Recent Advances in Flatology." *New England Journal of Medicine* (June 1980):100.

CHAPTER 6. WHAT TO DO ABOUT HEARTBURN

Dubey, P., K. R. Sundram, and S. Nundy. "Effect of Tea on Gastric Acid Secretion." *Digestive Diseases and Sciences* 1984; 29(3): 202–206.

Farinati, Fabio, et al. "Effects of N-Acetyle-L-Cysteine in Patients with Chronic Atrophic Gastritis and Nonulcer Dyspepsia: A Phase III Pilot Study." *Current Therapeutic Research* 1997; 58(10):724–733.

Feldman, M. and C. Barnett. "Relationship between the Acidity and Osmolarity of Popular Beverages and Reported Postprandial Heartburn." *Gastroenterology* 1995; 108:125.

Grande, Luis, M.D., et al. "Effects of Red Wine on 24-hour Esophageal pH and Pressures in Healthy Volunteers." *Digestive Diseases and Sciences* 1997; 42(6):1189–1192.

Iacono, Giuseppe, M.D., et al. "Gastroesophageal Reflux and Cow's Milk Allergy in Infants: A Prospective Study." *Journal of Allergy and Clinical Immunology* 1996; 97:822–7.

May, Burkard, et al. "Efficacy of a Fixed Peppermint Oil/Caraway Oil Combination in Non-Ulcer Dyspepsia." Arzneim.-Forsch/Drug Res. 1996; 46 (II);1149–1153.

Schönfeld, J.V., et al. "Oesophageal Acid and Salivary Secretion: Is Chewing Gum a Treatment Option for Gastro-oesophageal Reflux?" *Digestion* 1997; 58:111–114.

Thomas, W. E. G. "Duodeno-gastric Reflux—A Common Factor in Pathogenesis of Gastric and Duodenal Ulcer." *The Lancet* (November 19, 1980): 1166–1168.

CHAPTER 7. CAUSES AND TREATMENTS OF CONSTIPATION

Donaldson, A. N., M.D. "Relation of Constipation to Intestinal Intoxication." *Journal of the American Medical Association.* (March 25, 1992): 884–885.

Graham, David Y., M.D., S. E. Moser, M.D., and M. K. Estes. "The Effect of Bran on Bowel Function in Constipation." *American Journal of Gastroenterology* 1982; 77(9):599–603.

Harvey, R. F., E. E. Pomare, and K. W. Heaton. "Effects of Increased Dietary Fibre on Intestinal Transit." *The Lancet* (June 9, 1973): 1278–1280.

Iacono, Giuseppe, M.D., et al. "Intolerance of Cow's Milk and Chronic Constipation in Children." *New England Journal of Medicine* 1998; 339:1100–4.

Kreek, M. J., et al. "Naloxone, A Specific Opioid Antagonist, Reverses Chronic Idiopathic Constipation." *The Lancet* (February 5, 1983).

Marlett, J. A., J. L. Slavin, and P. M. Brauer. "Comparison of Dye and Pellet Gastrointestinal Transit Time during Controlled Diets Differing in Protein and Fiber Levels." *Digestive Diseases and Sciences* 1981; 26(3):208–213.

Keeling, W. F. and B. J. Martin. "Gastrointestional Transit During Mild Exercise." *Journal of Applied Physiology* 1987; 63:978–981.

CHAPTER 8. EASY TREATMENTS FOR DIARRHEA

Ament, Marvin E., M.D. "Malabsorption of Apple Juice and Pear Nectar in Infants and Children: Clinical Implications." *Journal of the American College of Nutrition* 1996; 15(5): 26S–29S.

De la Motte, S., et al. "Doppelglind-Vergleich Zwischen einem Alfelperktin/Kamillenextrakt-Praparat und Plazebo bei Kindern mit diarrhoe" *Arzneim.-forsch./Drug Res* 1997; 47(11):1247–1249.

Fernandes, C. F., K. M. Shahani, and M. A. Amer. "Control of Diarrhea by Lactobacilli." *Journal of Applied Nutrition* 1988; 40(1).

Gorbach, Sherwood L., M.D. "Efficacy of *Lactobacillus* in Treatment of Acute Diarrhea." *Nutrition Today Supplement* 1996; 31(6):19S–23S.

Gruskay, F. L., M.D. and R. E. Cooke, M.D. "The Gastrointestinal Absorption of Unaltered Protein in Normal Infants and in Infants Recovering from Diarrhea." *Pediatrics* 1954; 16:763–767.

Haffeejee, I. E. "Effect of Oral Folate on Duration of Acute Infantile Diarrhoea." Letter to *The Lancet* (August 6, 1988):334–335.

Journal of the American Medical Association. "Treatment of Chronic Diarrhea with Hydrochloric Acid." *JAMA* (July 1902):55.

Lifshitz, Fima, M.D. "Weaning foods . . . The role of Fruit Juice in the Diets of Infants and Children. *Journal of the American College of Nutrition* 1996; 15(5):1S–3S.

Mehta, M. N. and S. Subramaniam. "Comparison of Rice Water, Rice Electrolyte Solution, and Glucose Electrolyte Solution in the Management of Infantile Diarrhoea." *The Lancet* (April 1986):843–845.

Sazawal, S. R. E., et al. "Zinc Supplementation in Young Children with Acute Diarrhea in India." *New England Journal of Medicine* 1995; 333(13):839–843.

Vanderhoof, Jon A., M.D., et al. "Use of Soy Fiber in Acute Diarrhea in Infants and Toddlers." *Clinical Pediatrics* (March 1997):135–139.

Vannatta, J. B., M.D., D. Adamson, and Ken Mullican. "Blastocystis Hominis Infection Presenting as Recurrent Diarrhea." *Annals of Internal Medicine* 1985;102(4):495–496.

CHAPTER 9. KEYS TO OVERCOMING DIVERTICULAR DISEASE

Brodribb, A. J. M. "Treatment of Symptomatic Diverticular Disease with a High-Fibre Diet." *The Lancet* (March 16, 1977):664–666.

Corry, D. C., M.D. "Milk in Diverticula of Colon." *British Medical Journal* (April 1963): 929–930.

Findlay, J. M., et al. "Effects of Unprocessed Bran on Colon Function in Normal Subjects and in Diverticular Disease." *The Lancet* (February 2, 1974):146–149.

Gear, J. S. S., et al. "Symptomless Diverticular Disease and Intake of Dietary Fibre." *The Lancet* (March 10, 1979):511–514.

Ornstein, M. H., et al. "Are Fibre Supplements Really Necessary in Diverticular Disease of the Colon? A Controlled Clinical Trial." *British Medical Journal* 1981; 282:1353–1356.

Painter, Neil S. "Milk and Diverticulosis." Letter to *British Medical Journal* (May 1963): 1290.

Painter, Neil S., A. Z. Almeida, and K. W. Colebourne. "Unprocessed Bran in Treatment of Diverticular Disease of the Colon." *British Medical Journal* 1972; 2:137–140.

Painter, Neil S. and Denis P. Burkitt. "Diverticular Disease of the Colon: A Deficiency Disease of Western Civilization." *British Medical Journal* 1971; 2:450–454.

CHAPTER 10. EASY PREVENTION AND CURE OF HEMORRHOIDS

Arabi, Y., et al. "Trial of High Fibre Diet or Local Treatment for Patients with Heamorrhoids." Abstract in *British Society of Gastroenterology:* A987.

Dam, H., et al. "Gall Bladder Problems." *Acta Physiology Scandinavia* 1956; 36:329.

Hodgen, R. E., et al. *American Journal of Clinical Nutrition* 1962; 11(180):187.

Perez-Maranda, M., et al. "Effect of Fiber Supplements on Internal Bleeding Hemorrhoids." *Heapto-Gastroenterology* 1996; 43:1504–1507.

CHAPTER 11. NATURAL ANSWERS FOR INFLAMMATORY BOWEL DISEASE

Breuer, R. I., et al. "Short Chain Fatty Acid Rectal irrigation for Left-Sided Ulcerative Colitis: A Randomised, Placebo Controlled Trial." *Gut* 1997; 40:485–491.

Cattaneo. M., et al. "High Prevalence of Hyperhomocysteinemia in Patients with Inflammatory Bowel Disease: a Pathogenic Link with Thromboembolic Complications?" *Thromboembolitic Haemostology* 80:542–5 (1998).

Darroch, C. J., R. M. R. Barnes, and J. Dawson. "Circulating Antibodies to *Saccharomyces Cerevisiae* (Bakers'/Brewers' Yeast) in Gastrointestinal Disease." *Journal of Clinical Pathology* 1999; 52:47–53.

Dvorak, Ann M. "Vitamin A in Crohn's Disease." Letter to *The Lancet* (June 14, 1980): 1303–1304.

Ellestad-Sayed, J. J., et al. "Pantothenic Acid, Coenzyme A, and Human Chronic Ulcerative and Granulomatous Colitis." *American Journal Clinical Nursing* 1976; 29:1333–1338.

Hague, A., B. Singh, and C. Paraskeva. "Butyrate Acts as a Survival Factor for Colonic Epithelial Cells: Further Fuel for the In Vivo versus in Vitro Debate." *Gastroenterology* 1997; 112(3): 1036–1039.

Hallak, Silkoff K., A. Yegena, et al. "Consumption of Refined Carbohydrate by Patients with Crohn's Disease in Tel Aviv-Yafo." *Postgraduate Medical Journal* 1980; 56:842–6.

Hillier, K., et al. "Incorporation of Fatty Acids from Fish Oil and Olive Oil into Colonic Mucosal Lipids and Effects upon Eicosanoid Synthesis in Inflammatory Bowel Disease." *Gut* 1991; 32:1151–1155.

Katschinski, B., et al. "Smoking and Sugar Intake are Separate but Interactive Risk Factors in Crohn's Disease." *Gut* 1988; 29:1202–1206.

Mackie, Thomas T., M.D. "Food Allergy in Ulcerative Colitis." *Journal of the American Dietetic Association* 1938; 14:177–180.

Malin, Merja, et al. "Promotion of IgA Immune Response in Patients with Crohn's Disease by Oral Bacteriotherapy with *Lactobacillus* GG." *Annals of Nutritional Metabolism* 1996; 40:137–145.

Matsui, Toshiyuki, M.D. "Zinc Deficiency in Crohn's Disease" *Journal of Gastroenterology* 1998; 33:924–925.

Nakamura, T., et al. "Zinc Clearance Correlates with Clinical Severity of Crohn's Disease: A Kinetic Study." *Digestive Diseases and Sciences* 1988; 33(12):1520–1524.

Reif, S., et al. "Pre-illness Dietary Factors in Inflammatory Bowel Disease." *Gut* 1997; 40: 754–760.

Rowe, A. H., M.D., A. Rowe, Jr., M.D., and K. Uyeyama, M.D. "Regional Enteritis—Its Allergic Aspects." *Gastroenterology* 1953; 23:554–571.

Sandborn, William J., M.D., et al. "Transdermal Nicotine for Mildly to Moderately Active Ulcerative Colitis." *Annals of Internal Medicine* 1997; 126:364–371.

Sandha, G. S., et al. "Effect of Smoking on the Clinical Relapse of Inflammatory Bowel Disease (IBD) Before, During and After Pregnancy." *Canadian Journal of Gastroenterology* 1997; 11(Supple A): 55A.

Schumert, R., M.D., J. Towner, and R. D. Zipser, M.D. "Role of Eicosanoids in Human and Experimental Colitis." *Digestive Diseases and Sciences* 1988; 33(3):58S–64S.

Skogh, M., T. Sundquist, and C. Tagesson. "Vitamin A in Crohn's Disease." Letter to *Lancet* (April 5, 1980):766.

Stoll, R., et al. "Functional Defect of Zinc Transport in Patients with Crohn's Disease." *Hepato-Gastroenterology* 1987; 34:178–181.

Tiomny, E., et al. "Serum Zinc and Taste Acuity in Tel-Aviv Patients with Inflammatory Bowel Disease." *American Journal of Gastroenterology* 1982; 77(2):101.

CHAPTER 12. NEW TREATMENTS FOR PEPTIC ULCER AND INFLAMED STOMACH

Aiba, Yuji M.T., et al. "Lactic Acid-Mediated Suppression of *Helicobacter Pylori* by the Oral Administration of *Lactobacillus Salivarius* as a Probiotic in Gnotobiotic Murine Model." *Am J. Gastroenterol* 1998; 93:2097–2101.

Aldoori, Walid H., et al. "Prospective Study of Diet and the Risk of Duodenal Ulcer in Men." *American Journal of Epidemiology* 1997; 145(1):42–50.

Boutsen, Y., et al. "Antacid-Induced Osteomalacia." *Clinical rheumatology* 1996; 15(1):75–80.

Cave, David R. "*Helicobacter Pylori* and Its Interaction with Chief and Parietal Cells." *Yale Journal of Biology and Medicine* 1996; 69:91–98.

Corrado, G., et al. "Positive Association between Helicobacter Pylori Infection and Food Allergy in Children." *Scandinavian Journal of Gastroenterology* 33(11):1135–9 (1998)

Escolar, G., and O. Bulbena. "Zinc Compounds, a New Treatment in Peptic Ulcer." *Drugs Experimental Clinical Research* 1989; XV(2):83–89.

Figura, N., et al., and Parente, F., et al. "Nongastric Diseases Related to H. Pylori Infections. Five Abstracts." *Gut* 1996; 39 (Suppl 2): A93.

Glavin, G. B. and A. M. Hall. "Brain-Gut Relationships: Gastric Mucosal Defense Is Also Important." *Acta Physiologica Hungarica* 1992; 80:107–15.

Halter, F. and R. K. Zetterman. "Long-Term Effects of *Helicobacter Pylori* Infection on Acid and Pepsin Secretion." *Yale Journal of Biology and Medicine* 1996; 69:99–104.

Heffernon, E. W., M.D., E. D. Keifer, M.D., and M. L. Tracey, M.D. "Benign Gastric Ulcers Occurring in the Presence of Aghlorhydria: Report of Two Cases." *New England Journal of Medicine* (October 1949):604.

Kabir, A. M. A., et al. "Prevention of *Helicobacter Pylori* Infection by Lactobacilli in a Gnotobiotic Murine Model." *Gut* 1997; 41:49–55.

Madinier, Isabelle M., T. M. Fosse, and R. A. Monteil. "Oral Carriage of *Helicobacter Pylore:* A Review." *Journal of Periodontology* 1997; 68:2–6.

Minddel, Joel S., M.D. and E. William Rosenberg, M.D. "Is *Helicobacter Pylori* of Interest to Ophthalmologists?" *Ophthalmology* 1997; 104(11): 1729–30.

Nagaoka, Masato, et al. "Anti-Ulcer Effects of Lactic Acid Bacteria and Their Cell Wall Polysaccharides." *Biological and Pharmaceutical Bulletin* 1994; 17(8):1012–1017.

NIH Consensus Conference. "*Helicobacter pylori* in Peptic Ulcer Disease." *Journal of the American Medical Association* 1994; 272(1):65–69.

Rodríguez, Luis A. García, Mari-Ann Wallander, and Bruno H. Ch. Stricker. "The Risk of Acute Liver Injury Associated with Cimetidine and Other Acid-Suppressing Anti-Ulcer Drugs." *Journal of Clinical Pharmacology* 1997; 43:183–188.

Salim, A. S. "A Possible New Approach to the Problem of Refractory Peptic Ulceration, a Role for Free Radical Scavengers?" *Scottish Medical Journal* 1991; 36:19–20.

Salim, A. S. "Oxygen-Derived Free Radicals and the Prevention of Duodenal Ulcer Relapse: A New Approach." *American Journal of Medical Science* 1990; 300:1–6.

Siegel, J., M.D. "Immunologic Approach to the Treatment and Prevention of Gastrointestinal Ulcers." *Annals of Allergy* (January 1977); 38:27–29.

Sivam, Gowsala P., et al. "*Helicobacter pylori—In vitro* Susceptibility to Garlic *(Allium Sativum)* extract." *Nutrition and Cancer* 1997; 27(2):118–121.

Weiner, H. and A.P. Shapiro. "Is *Helicobacter Pylori* Really *the* Cause of Gastroduodenal Disease?" *Quality Journal of Medicine* 1998; 91:707–711.

Chapter 13. Healing Gallbladder Disease

Breneman, J. C., M.D. "Allergy Elimination Diet As the Most Effective Gallbladder Diet." *Annals of Allergy* 1968; 20:83–87.

British Medical Journal. "Gall Stone Dissolution in Man Using an Essential Oil Preparation." *British Medical Journal* (January 1979):24.

Capper, W. M., et al. "Gallstones, Gastric Secretion, and Flatulent Dyspepsia." *The Lancet* (February 25, 1967): 413–415.

Dorvil, N. P., et al. "Taurine Prevents Cholestasis Induced by Lithocholic Acid Sulfate in Guinea Pigs." *American Journal of Clinical Nutrition* 1983; 37: 221–232.

Frahm, Ann E., with David J. Frahm. *A Cancer Battle Plan.* Colorado Springs, CO: Pinon Press, 1992.

Fravel, R. C., M.D. "The Occurrence of Hypochlorhydria in Gall-Bladder Disease." *American Journal of Medical Science* 1920; 159:512–517.

Ginter, Emil. "Cholesterol: Vitamin C Controls Transformation to Bile Acids." *Science* (February 1973) 179:702–706.

Jenkins, S. A. "Vitamin C and Gallstone Formation: A Preliminary Report." *Specialia* 1977; 15(12):1616–1617.

Mingrone, G., A. V. Greco, and S. Passi. "The Possible Role of Free Fatty Acids in the Pathogenesis of Cholesterol Gallstones in Man." *Biochimica et. Biopphysica Acta* 1983; 751:138–144.

Necheles, H., M.D., et al. "Allergy of the Gall Bladder: A Study Using the Graham-Cole Test and the Leucopenic Index." *American Journal of Digestive Diseases* 1940; 7(6):238–241.

Pixley, Fiona and J. Mann. "Dietary Factors in the Aetiology of Gall Stones: A Case Control Study." *Gut* 1988; 29:1511–1515.

Scragg, R. K. R., A. J. McMichael, and P. A. Baghurst. "Diet, Alcohol, and Relative Weight in Gall Dtone Disease: A Case-Control Study." *Scottish Medical Journal* (April 1984); 288: 1113–1119.

Thornton, J. R., P. M. Emmett, and K. W. Heaton. "Diet and Gall Stones: Effects of Refined and Unrefined Carbohydrate Diets on Bile Cholesterol Saturation and Bile Acid Metabolism." *Gut* 1983; 24:2–6.

Toouli, J., et al. "Gallstone Dissolution in Man Using Cholic Acid and Lecithin." *The Lancet* (December 6, 1975):1124–1126.

Walzer, M., M.D., et al. "The Allergic Reaction in the Rhesus Monkey: Experimental Studies in the Rhesus Monkey." *Gastroenterology* 1943; 19: 565–561.

Worthington, H. V., et al. "A Pilot Study of Antioxidant Intake in Patients with Cholesterol Gallstones" *Nutrition* 1997; 13(2):118–127.

CHAPTER 14. IRRITABLE BOWEL SYNDROME AND OTHER CAUSES OF INTESTINAL PAIN

Bijileveld, Charles, M.D., et al. "Excessive Fruit Juice Consumption: How Can Something That Causes Failure to Thrive Be Associated with Obesity?" *Pediatrics* 1997; 99:15–21.

Colon, A. R., M.D. and J. S. Dipalma, M.D. "Colic." *American Family Physician* 1989; 40(6): 122–124.

D'Eufemia, P., et al. "Abnormal Intestinal Permeability in Children with Autism." *Acta Paediatrica* 1996; 85:1076–9.

Dieterich, W., et al. "Autoantibodies to Tissue Transglutaminase As Predictors of Celiac Disease." *Gastroenterology* 1998; 115:1317–1321.

Felding, John F., M.D. "Detailed History and Examination Assist Positive Clinical Diagnosis of the Irritable Bowel Syndrome." *Journal of Clinical Gastroenterology* 1983; 5:495–497.

Fischer, Howard, M.D. "Cow Milk Protein As a Cause of Infantile Colic." Letter to *The Journal of Pediatrics* (June 1989).

Fukudo, S., et al. "Brain-Gut Interactions in Irritable Bowel Syndrome: Physiological and Psychological Aspect." *Nippon Rinsho—Japanese Journal of Clinical Medicine* 1992; 50(11): 2703–11.

Hoekstra, J. H., et al. "Fruit Juice Malabsorption, Not Only Fructose." *Acta Pediatrician* 1995: 1241–44.

Hemmings, W. A. and E. W. Williams. "Antigen Absorption by the Gut." *The Lancet* (September 30, 1978):715.

Hemmings, W. A. and E. W. Williams. "Transport of Large Breakdown Products of Dietary Proteins Through the Gut Wall." *Gut* 1978; 19(8):715–723.

Jacob, S., et al. "Exclusion Diet in Diarrhoeal Irritable Bowel Syndrome—Our Experience in Forty Patients." *Irish Journal of Medical Science* 1996; 165(Suppl4):11.

Kellow, J. E., et al. "Effects of Acute Psychologic Stress on Small-Intestinal Motility in Health and the Irritable Bowel Syndrome." *Scandanavian Journal Gastroenterology* 1992; 27:53–58.

Lindberg, Lothe L. "Cow's Milk Whey Protein Elicits Symptoms of Infantile Colic in Colicky Formula-Fed Infants: A Double-Blind Crossover Study." *Pediatrics* 1989; 83:262–266.

Liu, Jenn-Hua, et al. "Enteric-Coated Peppermint-Oil Capsules in the Treatment of Irritable Bowel Syndrome: A Perspective, Randomized Trial." *Gastroenterol* 1997; 32:765–768.

Lust, K. D., et al. "Maternal Intake of Cruciferous Vegetables and Other Foods in Colic Symptoms in Exclusively Breastfed Infants." *Journal of the American Dietetic Association* 1996; 91(1):46–48.

Niec, Anna M., et al. "Are Adverse Food Reactions Linked to Irritable Bowel Syndrome?" *American Journal of Gastroenterology* 1998; 93:2184–2190.

Nutrition Review. "Is Colic in Infants Associated with Diet?" Editorial in *Nutrition Review* 1988; 48(11):374–375.

Pettler, M. H., M.D., et al. "Peppermint Oil for Irritable Bowel Syndrome: A Critical Review and Metaanalysis." *American Journal of Gastroenterology* 1998; 93(7):1131–35.

Rumessen, J. J. and E. Gudmand-Hoyer. "Functional Bowel Disease: Malabsorption and Abdominal Distress After Ingestion of Fructose, Sorbitol, and Fructose-Sorbitol Mixtures." *Gastroenterology* 1988: 95:694–700.

Sasaki, D., et al. "Psychosomatic Treatment of Irritable Bowel Syndrome." *Nippon Rinsho—Japanese Journal of Clinical Medicine* 1992; 50(11):2758–63.

Weaver, L. T. "Soy-Based Infant Milk Formulas and Passive Intestinal Permeability." Letter to *The Lancet*. (May 6, 1989):1023.

"What's Gastroprotective? Chili Powder." *Modern Medicine* 1995; 63:11.

CHAPTER 15. INTESTINAL INVADERS: PARASITES

Archer, D. L. and W. H. Glinsmann, M.D. "Intestinal Infection and Malnutrition Initiate Acquired Immune Deficiency Syndrome (AIDS)." *Nutrition Research* 1984; 5:9–19.

Crook, W. G. *Chronic Fatigue Syndrome and the Yeast Connection.* Jackson, TN: Professional Books, 1992.

Das, U. N. "Rectal Infusion of Bacterial Preparations for Intestinal Disorders." Letter to *The Lancet* (December 24/31, 1983): 1494–1495.

Emergency Medicine. "Stalking the Elusive Giardia Lamblia." *Emergency Medicine* (August 1984): 150–153.

Galland, L. and H. Bueno. "Advances in Laboratory Diagnosis of Intestinal Parasites." *American Clinical Laboratory* 1989; 18–19.

Levison, Matthew E., M.D. "How to Diagnose and Treat Diarrhea Due to Enteric Pathogens." *Medical Times* (March 1981): 47–53.

Nanda, R., B. S. Anand, and U. Baveja. "Entamoeba Histolytica Cyst Passers: Clinical Features and Outcomes in Untreated Subjects." *The Lancet* (August 11, 1984): 301–303.

Scott, Shirley, M.D. "Sources of Parasitic Infections." *CRIF Newsletter* (December 1986): 21–22.

Wolfe, Martin S. "Symptomatology, Diagnosis, and Treatment." In *Giardia & Giardioas: Biology, Pathogenesis, & Epidemiology.* New York and London: Premium Press, 1984.

CHAPTER 16. THE CANDIDA-RELATED COMPLEX

Collins, E. B. and P. Hardt. "Inhibition of Candida Albicans by Lactobacillus *Acidophilus.*" *Journal of Dairy Science* 1980; 63(5):830–832.

Crook, William G., M.D. *The Yeast Connection: A Medical Breakthrough.* 2nd ed. Jackson, TN: Professional Books, 1984.

De Schepper, Luc. *Candida.* Santa Monica, CA: Luc De Schepper, 1986.

Kennedy, Michael J. and Paul A. Volz. "Ecology of Candida Albicans Gut Colonisation: Inhibition of Candida Adhesion, Colonization, and Dissemination from the Gastrointestinal Tract by Bacterial Antagonism." *Infection and Immunity* 1985; 49(3):654–663.

Mathur, S., et al. "Anti-Ovarian and Anti-Lymphocyte Antibodies in Patients with Chronic Vaginal Candidiasis." *Journal of Reproductive Immunology* 1980; 2: 247.

Nystatin Multicenter Study Group. "Therapy of Candidal vaginitis: the effect of eliminating intestinal candida." *American Journal of Obstetric Gynecology* 1986; 155:561.

Position statements. "Candidiasis Hypersensitivity Syndrome." Approved by the Executive Committee of the American Academy of Allergy and Immunology. *Journal of Allergy and Clinical Immunology* 1986; 38(2):271–273.

Schinfeld, J. S. "PMS and Candidiasis: Study Explores Possible Link." *Female Patient* (July 1987): 66.

Slutsky, B., J. Buffo, and D. R. Soll. "High-Frequency Switching of Colony Morphology in Candida Albicans." *Science* 20: 666–668.

Sobell, Jack D., M.D. "Recurrent Vulvovaginal Candidiasis: A Prospective Study of the Efficacy of Maintenance Ketoconazole Therapy." *New England Journal of Medicine* 1985; 315(23):1455–8.

Tait, M. J. "Mustard Vegetables for Candida Immunity." Letter to *New Zealand Medical Journal* 98 (1985). Reviewed in *International Clinical Nutrition* July 1986; *Review* 8(3):143.

Trowbridge, J. P., M.D. and M. Walker. *The Yeast Syndrome.* New York: Bantam, 1986.

Truss, C. Orian, M.D. "Metabolic Abnormalities in Patients with Chronic Candidiasis: The Acetaldehyde Hypothesis." *Journal of Orthomolecular Psychiatry* 15(2): 67–93.

Truss, C. Orian, M.D. "The Role of Candida Albicans in Human Illness." Reprinted from *Journal of Orthomolecular Psychiatry* 1981; 10(4):1–3.

Truss, C. Orian, M.D. "Tissue Injury Induced by Candida Albicans: Mental and Neurologic Manifestations." *Journal of Orthomolecular Psychiatry* 1978; 7(1):17.

CHAPTER 17. THE INTESTINAL TRACT AND SERIOUS DISEASE

Colorectal Cancer

Calder P. C., et al. "Dietary Fish Oil Supresses Human Colon Tumor Growth in Athymic Mice." *Clinical Science* 94:303–311 (1998).

Corpet, E. D., et al. "Cooked Casein Promotes Colon Cancer in Rats, May Be Because of Mucosal Abrasion." *Cancer Letters* 114:89–90 (1997).

Grahan, S., et al. "Alimentary Factors in the Epidemiology of Gastric Cancer." *Cancer* 30:927–938 (1972).

Howe, G. R., et al. "The Relationship Between Dietary Fat Intake and Risk of Colorectal Cancer: Evidence from the Combined Analysis of 13 Case-Control Studies." *Cancer Causes and Control* 8:215–228 (1997).

Ireland, A. P., et al. "Gastric Juice Protects Against the Development of Esophageal Adenocarcinoma in the Rat." *Annals of Surgery* 224(3):358–371 (1996).

Leyton, E. "Nutritional Intervention in Carcinoma of the Colon." *Alternative & Complementary Therapies* Sept/Oct.:322–327 (1995).

Probst-Hensch, N. M., et al. "Meat Preparation and Colorectal Adenomas in a Large Sigmoidoscopy-Based Case-Control Study in California (United States)." *Cancer Causes and Control* 8:175–183 (1997).

Psathakis, D., et al. "Blood Selenium and Glutathione Peroxidase Status in Patients with Colorectal Cancer." *Diseases of Colon and Rectum* 41:328–335 (1998).

Russo, M. W., et al. "Plasma Selenium Levels and the Risk of Colorectal Adenomas." *Nutrition and Cancer* 28(2):125–129 (1997).

Slattery, M. L., et al. "Plant Foods and Colon Cancer: An Assessment of Specific Foods and Their Related Nutrients (United States)." *Cancer Causes and Control*:575–590 (1997).

Szilagyi, A. "Altered Colonic Environment, A Possible Predisposition to Colorectal Cancer and Colonic Inflammatory Disease." *Canadian Journal of Gastroenterology* 12(2): 133–146 (1998).

Tangrea, J., et al. "Serum Levels of Vitamin D Metabolites and the Subsequent Risk of Colon Cancer and Rectal Cancer in Finnish Men." *Cancer Causes and Control* 8:615–625 (1997).

Wu, A. H., et al. "Alcohol and Tobacco Use: Risk Factors for Colorectal Ademona and Carcinoma." *JNCI* 87(4):239–240 (1995).

Xue, L., et al. "Influence of Dietary Calcium and Vitamin D on Diet-Induced Epithelial Cell Hyperproliferation in Mice." *Journal of the National Cancer Institute* 91:176–181 (1999).

AIDS

Archer, D. L., et al. "Enteric Infection and Other Cofactors in AIDS." *Immunology Today* (1985).

Bower, M. "Diarrhea and AIDS." *Bulletin of Experimental Treatments for AIDS.* June (1997).

Bjarnason, I., et al. "Intestinal Inflammation, Ileal Structure and Function in HIV." *AIDS* 10:1385–1391 91996).

Greenberg, P. D., et al. "Treatment of Severe Diarrhea Caused by Cryptosporidium Parvum with Oral Bovine Immunoglobulin Concentrate in Patients with AIDS." *Journal of Immune Deficiency Syndromes and Human Retrovirology* 13:348–354 (1996).

Ramratnam, B., et al. "A Practical Approach to Managing Diarrhea in the HIV-Infected Person." *The AIDS Reader* 7(6):190–196 (1997).

Romeyn, M. *Nutrition and HIV: A New Model for Treatment.* Jossey-Bass, San Francisco. (1995).

Standish, L. J. "Alternative medicine in HIV/AIDS: Current state of the science and justification for research." (1996).

Yee, J., et al. "Gastrointestinal Manifestations of AIDS." *Gastroenterology Clinics of North America* 24(2):413–434 (1995)

CHAPTER 18: FINDING AND HEALING YOUR FOOD ALLERGIES

Bengtsson, U., L. A. Hanson, and S. Ahlstedt. "Survey of Gastrointestinal Reactions to Foods in Adults in Relation to Atopy, Presence of Mucus in the Stools, Swelling of Joints and Arthralgia in Patients with Gastrointestinal Reactions to Foods." *Clinical and Experimental Allergy* 1996; 2:1387–1394.

Bhna, Sami L., M.D. and Clifton T. Furukawa, M.D. "Food Allergy: Diagnosis and Treatment." Annals of *Allergy* (December 1983); 51:574–580.

Bischoff, S. C., A. Herrmann, and M. P. Manns. "Prevalence of Adverse Reactions to Food in Patients with Gastrointestinal Disease." *Allergy* 1996; 51:811–818.

Corrado, G., et al. "Positive Association Between *Helicobacter Pylori* Infection and Food Allergy in Children." *Scandinavian Journal of Gastroenterology* 1998; 33:1135–1139.

Finn, R. and H. N. Cohen. "Food Allergy: Fact or Fiction?" *The Lancet* 1978; 1(8061):426–428.

Golbert, T. M., M.D., R. Patterson, M.D., and J. J. Pruzansky. "Systemic Allergic Reactions to Ingested Antigens." *Journal of Allergy* 1989; 44(2):96–107.

Hamburger, Robert N., M.D. "Food Allergy: Confessions of an Agnostic: Overt to Covert." Bela Shick Lecture in *Annals of Allergy* (May 1988); 60:454–458.

Hemmings, W. A. "Food Allergy." Letter to *The Lancet* (March 18, 1978): 608.

Ingelfinger, F. J., M.D., F. C. Lowell, M.D., and W. Franklin, M.D. "Gastrointestinal Allergy." *New England Journal of Medicine* 1949; 241(8):301–308.

Klein, N. C., M.D., et al. "Eosinophilic Gastroenteritis." *Medicine* 1970; 49(4):299–319.

Mayron, Lewis W. "Portals of Entry—A Review." *Annals of Allergy* 1978; 40(6):399–403.

Metcalfe, Dean D., M.D., and Michael A. Kaliner, M.D. "What Is Food to One . . ." Editorial in *New England Journal of Medicine* 1984; 311(6):399–400.

Ring, Johannes. "Allergy and Modern Society: Does 'Western Life Style' Promote the Development of Allergies?" *International Archives of Allergy and Immunology* 1997; 113:7–10

Watt, J., J. R. Pincott and J. T. Harries. "Combined Cow's Milk Protein and Gluten-Induced Enteropathy: Common or Rare?" *Gut* 1983; 24:165–170.

Zioudrou, C., R. A. Streaty, and W. A. Klee. "Opioid Peptides Derived from Food Proteins: The Exorphins." *Journal of Biological Chemistry* 1979; 254(7):2446–2449.

CHAPTER 19. USING YOUR POWER TOOLS: DIGESTIVE ENZYMES

HCl

Andres, M. R., Jr., M.D., and J. R. Bingham, M.D. "Tubeless Gastric Analysis with a Radio-Telemetering Pill (Heidelberg capsule)." *C.M.A. Journal* 1970; 102:1087–1089.

Capper, W. M., et al. "Gallstones, Gastric Secretion and Flatulent Dyspepsia." *The Lancet* (February 25, 1967): 413–415.

Feldman, Mark, M.D. "The Mature Stomach: Still Pumping Out Acid?" *Journal of the American Medical Association* 1997; 278(8):681–2.

Findley, J. W., Jr., M.D., J. B. Kirsner, M.D., and W. L. Palmer, M.D. "Atrophic Gastritis: A Follow-up Study of 100 Patients." *Gastroenterology* 1950; 16:347.

Goodman, L. S. and A. G. Gillman (eds.). *The Pharmacological Basis of Therapeutics,* Fourth Edition. New York: Macmillan, 1996.

Ramsey, E. J., et al. "Epidemic Gastritis with Hypochlorhydria." *Gastroenterology* 1979; 78:1440–1457.

Sharp, George S. and H. William Fisher, M.D. "The Diagnosis and Treatment of Achlorhydria." *Journal of the American Geriatric Society* 1967; 15(8).

Sharp, George S. and H. William Fisher, M.D. "The Diagnosis and Treatment of Achlorhydria: Ten-Year Study." *Journal of the American Geriatric Society* 1967; 15(8):786–791.

Trey, G., et al. "Changes in Acid Secretion Over the Years: A 30-Year Longitudinal Study." *Journal of Clinical Gastroenterology* 1997; 25(3):499–502.

Pancreatic Enzymes

DiMagno, E. P., M.D., et al. "Fate of Orally Ingested Enzymes in Pancreatic Insufficiency." *New England Journal of Medicine* 1977; 296(3):1318–1322.

Gyr, K., M.D., O. Felsenfeld, M.D., and M. Zimmerli-Ning, M.D. "The Effect of Oral Pancreatic Enzymes on the Intestinal Flora of Protein-Deficient Vervet Monkeys Challenged with Vibrio Cholerae." *American Journal of Clinical Nutrition* 1978; 32:1592–1596.

New England Journal of Medicine. "The Ins and Outs of Oral Pancreatic Enzymes." *New England Journal of Medicine* 1977; 296(23):1347.

Singh, Manjit, M.D. "Effect of Thiamin Deficiency on Pancreatic Acinar Cell Function." *American Journal of Clinical Nutrition* 1982; 36:500–504.

Zioudrou, C., R. A. Streaty, and W. A. Klee. "Opioid Peptides Derived from Food Proteins: The Exorphins." *Journal of Biological Chemistry* 1979; 254(7):2446–2449.

Bile

Crosignani, Andrea, et al. "Clinical Pharmacokinetics of Therapeutic Bile Acids." *Clinical Pharmacokinetics* 1996; 5:333–358.

CHAPTER 20. DETOXIFICATION AND REBUILDING PROGRAMS

Anderson, K. E. "Influences of Diet and Nutrition on Clinical Pharmacokinetics." *Clinical Pharmacokinetics* 1988; 14:325–346.

Ben, M. "Is Detoxification a Solution to Occupational Health Hazards?" *National Safety News.* (May 1984).

Schnare, D. W., et al. "Evaluation of a Detoxification Regime for Fat Stored Xenobiotics." *Medical Hypothesis* 1982; 9:265–282.

Index

A

absorption, definition of, 9
acetaldehyde, 162–163
achlorhydria, 59
acidophilus. See Lactobacillus (L.) acidophilus
acid reflux. *See* gastroesophageal reflux
acute, definition of, 5
acute diarrhea, 78–81
acute gallbladder problems
  diet for, 132
  face acupoint for, 136
  symptoms of, 128
affirmations
  description and uses of, 6, 42, 43
  for detoxification and rebuilding, 214
  for diarrhea, 87
  for diverticular disease, 93
  for food allergy, 194
  for gallbladder, 136
  for gas, 56
  for heartburn, 64–65
  for hemorrhoids, 99
  for inflammatory bowel disease, 110
  for intestinal awareness and healing, 45–46
  for ulcers, 125
AIDS
  diarrhea and, 176–177
  digestion and, 177–178
  overview of, 174
  parasitic infection and, 150, 174–175
  systemic yeast infection and, 159
air, swallowing, and heartburn, 59
alcohol
  colorectal cancer and, 172
  digestion and overuse of, 10
  ulcers and, 116, 121
allantoin, 84

allergies
  delayed reaction, 185–186
  fiber sources and, 25
  friendly bacteria and, 34
  immediate, 185
  masked, 185–186
  See also food allergies
allergy elimination-reintroduction diet
  expectations for, 188–189
  food reactions during, 190
  foods to avoid, 186–187
  foods to eat, 187–188
  overview of, 186
  reintroduction phase, 189–190
allopathic, definition of, 1
aloe vera
  colitis and, 104
  constipation and, 74
  diarrhea and, 81
  diverticular disease and, 91
  gas and, 52
  heartburn and, 62
  hemorrhoids and, 97
  ulcers and, 115, 121, 123
alpha-galactosidase, 55
aluminum in antacids, 114–115
amaranth, 164
amino acid imbalance, symptoms of, 220
amoebic infection, 34, 149
anemia
  celiac disease and, 142
  severe colitis and, 102
  ulcers and, 114
anger and ulcers, 125
antacids
  chronic use of, 62, 173
  ulcers, inflammation of stomach, and, 114–115

CPSIA information can be obtained at www.ICGtesting.com
Printed in the USA
BVOW03s0637100614

355931BV00011B/290/P

9 780471 349624